Contents

Introduction

I am thrilled you are holding this book because it means you are thinking about making a positive change to your overall health.

My husband Mark and I started our keto journey in May 2018. Between the two of us, we effortlessly lost a total of 25kg (55lb/4 stone) in less than six months – and now happily maintain our target weight along with excellent BMIs. In addition, we enjoy a euphoric flow of consistent energy and mental clarity; all this from reducing our intake of carbohydrates and enjoying plenty of natural fat.

My story may be like yours; by the time I was in my late thirties, my jeans were several sizes bigger, I was often tired... and where had my cheekbones gone? If I needed to shift weight for special occasions, I would starve myself using calorie-restricted diets. But the weight always came back and brought another fat roll for company. Oh, the agony! As a lover of delicious food, this was a depressing and unsustainable way to live and I spiralled downward into misery.

When the concept of the ketogenic diet exploded around the globe (and it's not really a new concept at all – the ketogenic diet has been used by doctors for many years to effectively reduce seizures in children suffering from epilepsy), I absorbed it like a thirsty sponge.

'*Say whaaat?* I can have double cream in my coffee and enjoy steak and crispy chicken skin as long as I skip the bread? Umm ... yes please!'

I read about people dropping pounds, reducing medication for chronic conditions and even reversing type 2 diabetes – while eating steak, butter and bacon! It didn't take much to convince us: we were both on board.

Just short of a month after starting the keto lifestyle and fuelled by the incredible results we both experienced, I started blogging about the recipes I was making at home. Rich, fatty, delicious food – it almost felt 'naughty'. I say naughty because keto living is quite opposite to the UK government guidelines on nutrition.

These guidelines are largely based on an American physiologist named Ancel Keys and his Seven Countries Study back in the late 1950s, where he set out to prove the link between fat in the diet and heart disease. His published findings did not go unchallenged by many respected medical professionals, who criticized the study and pointed out some serious flaws. However, the guidelines stuck: the recommendation was to reduce fat in the diet and increase grains and carbohydrates. But here we are, fifty-plus years later – fatter and sicker than ever. One cannot help asking, 'Did we get it horribly wrong?'.

Within six months, my blog was nominated as one of the top eight culinary blogs in the UK (UK Blog Awards, 2019) and I realized I had a purpose, a responsibility. I am not a doctor, but I am a chef. I have now passionately embarked on a mission to show people that the keto lifestyle is not all about bacon, eggs and cheese; it's exciting, delicious, limitless and very sustainable long term.

Monya

Keto Kitchen

Delicious recipes for energy and weight loss

Monya Kilian Palmer

Photography by Maja Smend

KYLE BOOKS

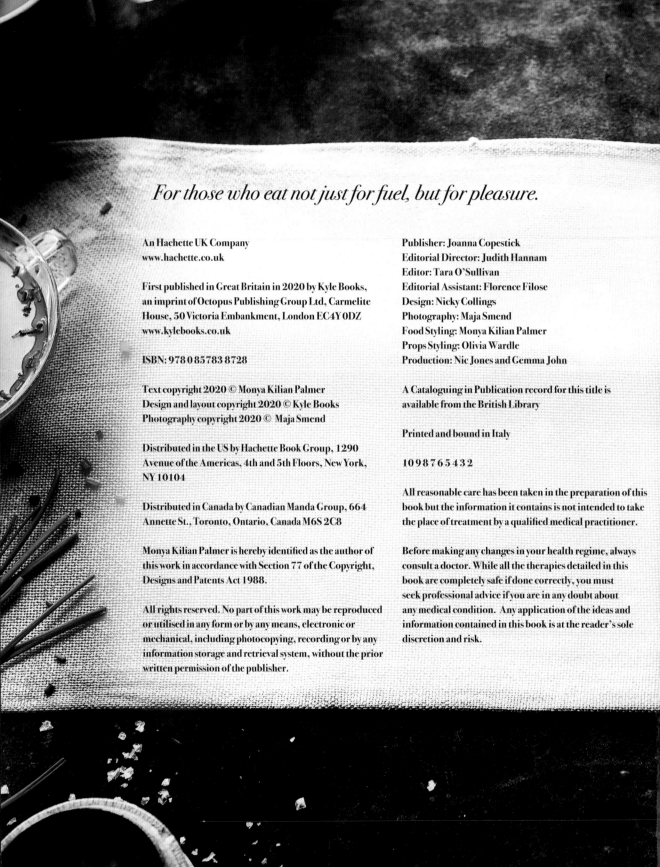

For those who eat not just for fuel, but for pleasure.

An Hachette UK Company
www.hachette.co.uk

First published in Great Britain in 2020 by Kyle Books,
an imprint of Octopus Publishing Group Ltd, Carmelite
House, 50 Victoria Embankment, London EC4Y 0DZ
www.kylebooks.co.uk

ISBN: 978 0 85783 8728

Distributed in the US by Hachette Book Group, 1290
Avenue of the Americas, 4th and 5th Floors, New York,
NY 10104

Distributed in Canada by Canadian Manda Group, 664
Annette St., Toronto, Ontario, Canada M6S 2C8

Publisher: Joanna Copestick
Editorial Director: Judith Hannam
Editor: Tara O'Sullivan
Editorial Assistant: Florence Filose
Design: Nicky Collings
Photography: Maja Smend
Food Styling: Monya Kilian Palmer
Props Styling: Olivia Wardle
Production: Nic Jones and Gemma John

A Cataloguing in Publication record for this title is
available from the British Library

Printed and bound in Italy

10 9 8 7 6 5 4 3 2

Keto Basics

'You want to keep the natural fats high, the protein moderate and the carbs low.'

The ketogenic diet is a lifestyle where your body uses fat, as opposed to carbohydrates, as its primary fuel. This happens when you reduce your intake of carbohydrates, forcing the body to tap into fat (both excess fat stored in the body and fat that is consumed) as an energy source. This natural, healthy state is referred to as 'nutritional ketosis', and is a result of a magical metabolic shift that takes place.

Once you understand the how and why, this lifestyle becomes easy and you will enjoy many wonderful health benefits along with the welcome side effect of weight loss.

Like everything in life, knowledge is power. A solid understanding of the three macro-nutrients (or macros) that make up the calories in your food is essential. These macros are carbohydrates, proteins and fats – and the most important thing is knowing which foods are high in carbohydrates so that you can avoid them. You want to keep the natural fats high, the protein moderate and the carbs low.

Fats

Fats should be carefully selected, but this is easy: just make sure they are natural fats. For example, enjoy a rib-eye steak fried in real butter, but steer clear of processed vegetable oils (such as sunflower oil and canola oil) and hydrogenated fat. (The production process of these oils will make your toes curl!)

Fat is also very satiating: your meals will be richer, tastier and keep you fuller for longer. It's likely that you will eat less at mealtimes or even skip meals altogether because you simply aren't hungry. And there is nothing wrong with skipping a meal; listen to your body and eat only when you are hungry, it's really that simple. It's the combination of these factors that makes this lifestyle so sustainable.

Many people combine the keto lifestyle with Intermittent Fasting. I am a huge fan of short-term fasting for many reasons and want to encourage you to research it further if you are up for the challenge. From my own experience, I rarely experience true hunger thanks to the nature of this lifestyle, so fasting is easy for me. It may also interest you that whether it's cardio or resistance training (both of which I love to do), I train far better on a fasted stomach! Try it for yourself and you will see that one does not 'need' carbohydrates to run for 40 minutes or weight train effectively.

When frying, I like to use lard, butter or coconut oil. Not only are these options tastier, but they are stable fats – and even your best-quality olive oil becomes somewhat unstable at very high temperatures. Not all fats are the

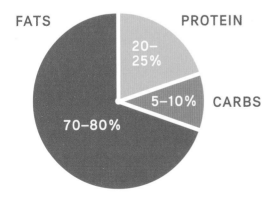

FATS — 70–80%

PROTEIN — 20–25%

CARBS — 5–10%

same – their molecular structures differ. Without boring you too much with the science, stable fats are fats that do not oxidize when heated at very high temperatures (e.g. when frying) and therefore do not produce free radicals. An imbalance of free radical activity in the body leads to oxidative stress, which damages cells over time and can lead to a range of very serious diseases.

Occasionally, I use odourless coconut oil when I do not want a 'coconut' flavour to dominate (especially in baking). If using this somewhat refined version doesn't sit well with you, use regular coconut oil.

Protein

Protein comes from meat, poultry, seafood, eggs and full-fat dairy. Protein breaks down to amino acids, which may be burned in a similar way to glucose as well as via the ketogenic pathway, so it's advised to consume adequate (but not excessive) protein. Protein is also essential as it will ensure the body doesn't break down lean muscle mass while the pounds are coming off.

Carbohydrates

Carbs should be kept as low as possible. You want to aim for no more than 20–30g (net) carbs per day (see page 11 for more about net carbs) and these should come from a wide variety of high-fibre, nutrient-packed vegetables. Not all vegetables are considered keto-friendly (and most fruits aren't either, due to their high sugar content), so it's imperative that you familiarize yourself with the keto-friendly food list on page 9.

Insulin

This is a good time to tell you a little bit about insulin. Insulin is a hormone produced in the pancreas that decides exactly how your body uses its fuel. It is commonly referred to as the 'fat-making hormone' – and rightly so. You see, when we eat carbohydrates, our blood sugar

rises, and insulin is released. It converts and stores some of that glucose as glycogen, but any excess is stored as body fat. Unless you are an athlete or a gym fanatic, you will gradually gain body fat for this exact reason.

On a low-carb diet, there are also minimal fluctuations in blood sugar, so you will no longer experience hunger, cravings, mood swings or fatigue.

Another interesting aspect is that spikes in blood glucose can irritate blood vessels (including arterial linings), causing inflammation. This can lead to arterial damage.

Processed Food

Many people start keto by sticking to the suggested macro breakdown (low carb, moderate protein, high fat) with little thought for the kind of food they are putting into their bodies. Low-carb pepperoni or store-bought mayonnaise may seem convenient, but those yummy processed meats often include glucose or dextrose (anything ending in 'ose' is a form of sugar) and a few other inflammatory nasties. And store-bought mayonnaise? Well, this is almost always made with vegetable oil. These are just two examples, but it's worth knowing that to experience the overall health benefits associated with the reduction of processed (inflammatory) foods, you should aim to – as much as possible – use fresh ingredients that you prepare yourself at home so you know exactly what has gone into your food.

Read the Label

Get into the habit of reading food labels. If there is anything that you don't recognize, put it back on the shelf and walk on. Reading labels will also reveal how many items contain hidden sugars.

Dairy

Many people remove dairy completely on their keto journey. I personally have no cows' milk intolerances and have had no issues including a moderate amount of dairy in my diet (e.g. double cream or full-fat cheese). Regular milk on the other hand (even full-fat milk) will contain much higher amounts of lactose and should be avoided.

Sweeteners

A large part of living keto is breaking the addiction to sugar. Addiction is a harsh word but it's true in this case. Research (through MRI studies) has shown that sugar leads to dopamine release in areas of the brain associated with motivation and reward – the same areas that respond to addictive drugs. Exposure starts at a young age.

Artificial sweeteners (like aspartame) rarely affect blood sugar but I like to keep them to a minimum because of claims I have read that they are to blame for a range of health problems. Furthermore, you may find it interesting to learn that artificial sweeteners may still create an insulin response (our brains are smart), so for me it's simply a case of 'where there's smoke, there's fire' with this one. I therefore stick to natural sweeteners like erythritol, xylitol* or stevia. These natural sweeteners are sugar polyols and have no impact on blood sugar for most people. Some people report digestive discomfort when using these natural sweeteners, so find one that works for you and remember that the ultimate goal is to break the addiction to sweet things altogether.

Xylitol is toxic to dogs. If you choose to use it, please keep your keto cupcakes far away from your pooches!

Alcohol

Here's what you need to know: beer, sweet wine and most mixers are high in carbohydrates. However, spirits like whisky or gin contain zero carbs. Essentially, this means that a few beers may temporarily throw you out of ketosis (the metabolic process where your body is burning fat for fuel), but a Scotch-and-soda may not. Alcohol is also very high in empty calories (it has no nutritional value) and while most of us don't count calories on keto, it's important to remember that alcohol is metabolized differently. In fact, it's metabolized immediately. I won't go into the science here, just know that consuming (even zero-carb) alcohol may delay your weight-loss journey; it's best kept for special occasions. It also goes without saying that consuming alcohol lowers inhibitions and you want to be thinking sharp when making food choices. More importantly, take care of your liver. That precious organ works so hard – don't give it more to deal with than it already must.

Supplements

Many people require electrolytes (sodium, potassium, magnesium) when they first start the keto lifestyle. The significant reduction of carbohydrates (and associated water loss in the early days) could lead to what is known as keto flu. Keto flu refers to a series of unpleasant side effects that some people experience in the first week or two. It's quite normal to experience headaches, fatigue and muscle cramps. Introducing an electrolyte supplement may remedy this, but I have personally never experienced any of these symptoms apart from a little fatigue in the first 48 hours (and my husband didn't experience any 'side effects' at all). Perhaps it's because I season our meals very well and always included a wide variety of nutrient-packed foods ... who knows? Anyway, these side effects are temporary and should not discourage you. Your body is responding to this metabolic shift (and possibly also experiencing a 'sugar detox'). Either way, I think it's a great indication that you are doing something right – so push through it, it will pass!

Those on medication where a fine electrolyte balance is required (e.g. calcium channel blockers for hypertension/high blood pressure), or those with kidney disease should seek medical advice before supplementing electrolytes.

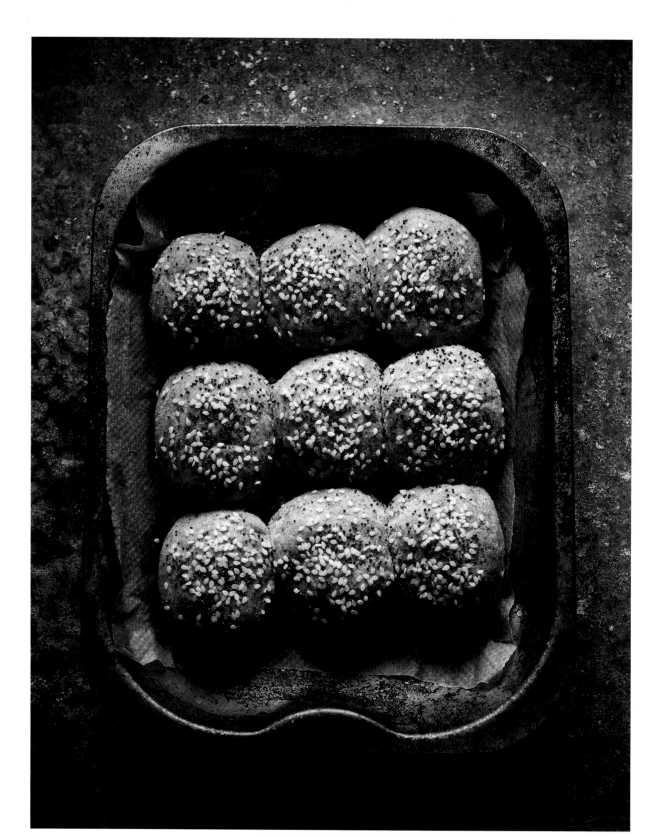

Keto-friendly Food

Below is a handy list of food that can be enjoyed on keto. Be mindful that, although many may be low in carbs, they still add up, so keep an eye on the amounts.

Fruit: Avocados, blackberries, blueberries, cranberries, lemons, limes, olives, raspberries, strawberries, tomatoes.

Fats: Animal fats (beef tallow/dripping, duck fat, goose fat, lard), avocado oil*, butter (grass-fed), cocoa butter, coconut oil, ghee, olive oil*, macadamia oil*, sesame oil* (*cold-pressed and not to be used for frying).

Fish and seafood: All fish and seafood can be enjoyed – opt for wild-caught and sustainable.

Meat, eggs and offal: All meat, eggs and offal can be enjoyed – opt for pasture-raised, free-range and organic. Do include offal (like kidneys or liver) in your diet – it is highly nutritious. Processed meats (like salami or pepperoni) should be for occasional consumption due to the unnecessary additives and hidden sugars present.

Nuts and seeds: All nuts and seeds (excluding rice) can be enjoyed but be wary as some are higher in carbs than others. Exercise a little restraint because it's easy to over-indulge when snacking on delicious nuts. Go easy on the nut flours too. While these are excellent substitutes to use in baking, the carbs can add up.

Vegetables: Artichokes, asparagus, aubergines, pak choi, broccoli, Brussels sprouts, cabbage, cauliflower, celeriac, celery, chillies, courgettes, cucumbers, fennel, garlic, green beans, kale, leeks, lettuce, mushrooms, okra, onions, peppers, pumpkin, radishes, rocket, spinach, watercress.

Herbs are great too and can be used to enhance flavour.

Ground spices, vinegar and mustard are all acceptable and I have never seen anything on the labels that troubles me. If in doubt, check the labels for hidden sugars.

Baking powder: Check the labels when using baking powder or bicarbonate of soda; most are gluten-free, but a quick check will help you make a better choice.

Foods to Avoid

All forms of sugar: This includes everything from regular table sugar to honey, and every other creative name companies are using as alternatives. Some examples include dextrose, maltose and corn syrup. Sugars that claim to be 'healthy' or 'natural' (like maple syrup or agave) are also bad news. **If it affects blood sugar, it should be avoided.** Remember that even milk contains lactose, so it's best replaced with a suitable alternative.

All forms of grains: This includes anything made with wheat flour (baked goods, bread, couscous, pasta) as well as any form of barley, millet, oats, rice and quinoa. Don't be fooled by 'gluten-free' products; these use rice, potato or tapioca flour and are often higher in carbs than wheat flour, creating even worse blood sugar spikes.

All starchy vegetables: This includes root vegetables like carrots, parsnips, potatoes, sweet potatoes and yams. Corn and butternut squash should also be avoided.

Fruit: Fruit can be very high in sugar (fructose, glucose and sucrose) and most should be avoided. See the keto-friendly food list opposite for low-sugar fruit options.

Legumes: All legumes are off-limits, and this includes beans, chickpeas, peas, peanuts, lentils and soy beans (this includes tofu or tempeh).

Starting the Keto Lifestyle

It can be overwhelming when you first start, but now that you have a little more knowledge and are not afraid of the commitment, the next part is easy!

Keep it simple when you start. Eat fatty cuts of meat like chicken, salmon, lamb or steak and enjoy these with your favourite vegetables from the keto-friendly food list (see page 9). Steer clear of any store-bought sauces or marinades and don't be afraid of natural, healthy fat. When you are ready and up for the challenge, try some of the more advanced recipes like the keto breads (see pages 18–21) or sweet treats (see pages 124–141) that use special ingredients.

Your time is precious but having an idea of what you will prepare in advance will make your life a lot easier. You can cleverly map out your weekly meals and this will help you shop smart and reduce waste.

Special Ingredients

There are a handful of 'special' ingredients that I would like to address. Most of my recipes include items you can get from your local supermarket or butcher. However there are some that you may not be familiar with, but can easily be sourced online.

Almond and coconut flours: When I refer to almond or coconut flour, I am not referring to meal, 'flurry' or any other version. Please only use the kind I specify for best results. It's also important to note that coconut flour is very different to almond flour and the two are not interchangeable in baking; they yield different results in texture, density and flavour.

Ground chia seeds and flaxseed: Some recipes call for ground chia and flaxseed. Do not try and grind whole seeds yourself unless you can achieve the very fine texture the store-bought ground kind offers. I keep all nut flours and ground seeds in a sealed container in the fridge to avoid possible rancidity.

Psyllium husk powder: Psyllium has fantastic thickening and binding qualities. When I refer to it in my recipes, it's the ground powder I use. Be careful when weighing it; a little under or over could make a significant difference.

Erythritol: Erythritol is my preferred natural sweetener. Where it's featured, it is the powdered/confectioners' (not granulated) kind I use. Sift it into your dry mix, as some brands 'clump' more than others. Erythritol has a slight 'cooling' effect on the palate and many people find that adding a few drops of liquid stevia balances this out. I have added this as an optional addition in the recipes where erythritol features in large quantities.

There is a huge psychological element to 'dieting' and none of us like to be told what we can't eat. I often tell people to focus on what we CAN eat and not on what we CAN'T. That mindset is so important and plays a huge role in keeping our eyes on the prize: health and energy (...and skinny jeans!)

About the Recipes

For the sake of convenience, the recipes in the book have been categorized into breakfasts, main meals, snacks and sweet treats. However, this doesn't necessarily mean you will be eating three meals a day and snacking in between. With a high-fat lifestyle, that is actually highly unlikely due to the reduction in hunger and cravings. Plus, there are no rules to say you can't have Salmon Eggs Benedict (page 26) for supper or leftover Lamb Shoulder (page 103) for breakfast. No judgement here ... I do it all the time!

The Nutritional Information

Unless otherwise stated, I have shown the macro breakdown per serving assuming the finished dish is divided into equal-sized servings. You may serve up differently, so use the nutritional information to guide your portion sizes. It's possible that your partner will want two chicken thighs while you are happy with one, or that you will want a larger steak than I have stated. It is impossible for me to anticipate every scenario, so I have stuck to moderate protein as keto suggests.

Food labels differ across the world. For simplicity's sake, I have shown only the information that we care about on keto – (net) carbohydrates, proteins and fats – as well as calories (for those who still monitor them).

Net Carbs

Some countries (like the USA) include dietary fibre in the total carb count on their food labels, which means that people should subtract this fibre to see what the 'net carbs' are. Net carbs are what we monitor on keto. Here in the UK, the carbs and dietary fibre are listed separately so the carbs we see are the net carbs. Without confusing you further (wherever you are in the world), I kept it simple; the carb counts shown in this book are the net carbs and therefore the carbs we should be monitoring.

Calculating the Nutritional Breakdown

The nutritional breakdown provided was calculated using the cloud-based software NUTRITICS®. NUTRITICS® is fully approved by the relevant Trading Standards organizations and is EU and FDA-compliant. I based the calculations on the trimmed weight of ingredients used in my recipes. Where erythritol (see page 10) was used in any of the recipes, I excluded its (non-impact) carbs from the displayed amount.

Cooking Tips

- Always read a recipe through before beginning, including the introduction. I usually include some information on why certain ingredients are used (especially in baking) and I often encourage you to use a little imagination and try different herbs or spices.

- Ensure your oven is preheated before cooking, and always check the temperature you should be aiming for, as fan-assisted ovens and conventional ovens differ.

- Chop and weigh your ingredients before you start cooking. This is referred to as *mis-en-place* (meaning 'everything in its place') in professional kitchens. A happy cook is an organized cook. This also allows you to do plenty of prep ahead of time, saving you more time to spend with your family or guests.

- I often add freshly chopped herbs or citrus zest to finish a dish after cooking. In most cases, these are essential flavour components, so please don't skip these garnishes.

- Regular coconut oil should be used in the recipes – and not the fractionated liquid kind.

- Where eggs are featured, I use free-range, large eggs. Sizes differ from store to store, though. If it helps, the whole eggs I used weighed around 57g (2oz) each.

- I refer to double cream in several recipes. In the UK this is a pourable cream with a higher fat content than regular cream. If you can't source it, use a high-fat, thickened cream and whisk it well before using to loosen it. Adding a teaspoon of water may help.

- An accurate digital kitchen scale is vital. Mine cost less than £10 and I use it a hundred times a week. Also, remember to zero your scale after placing the bowl on top, as well as in between adding each ingredient.

- When I refer to teaspoon or tablespoon measurements, these should be measured using standard, universal measuring spoons – and they should be levelled (not heaped) when using dry ingredients.

- Lastly, I hope you have a good-quality knife that you sharpen daily. If you cry when you cut onions, your knife needs sharpening: a blunt knife will crush the cell walls of the onion, releasing irritants, whereas a sharp knife will cleanly slice through the onion. A blunt or poor-quality knife is also far more dangerous as it will require more pressure to slice and this increases the risk of slipping and harming you. Now you know ...!

Happy cooking!

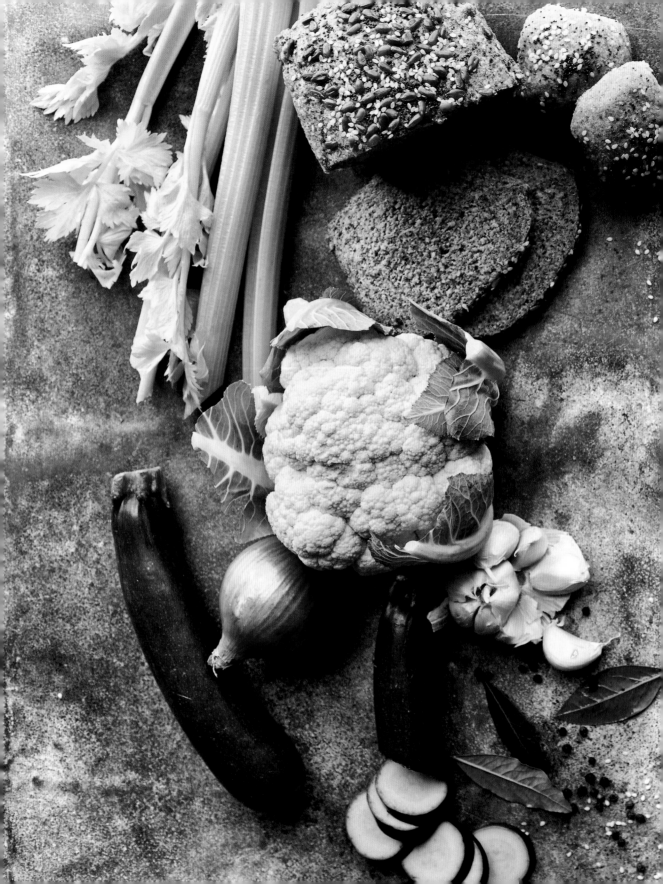

Broths,
Breads
& Bases

Beef Bone Broth

A cup of seasoned beef bone broth is a delicious, refreshing and surprisingly filling meal. I use an inexpensive pressure cooker to cook roasted bones. One batch makes approximately 2.5 litres (4½ pints) of the good stuff, so portion as needed and freeze in batches. This is a favourite of mine if I am doing some light fasting. A generous addition of salt stirred in at the end will finish each cup perfectly. If you have any herbs (like chives) to hand, they add lovely fresh top notes. *Pictured on page 2.*

9–10 SERVINGS | **10m** PREP TIME | **3hrs** COOK TIME | **12hrs** CHILLING TIME

2.5kg (5lb 8oz) beef bones (from your butcher)

2 celery stalks, roughly chopped

1 large onion, roughly chopped

3 garlic cloves

1 teaspoon whole black peppercorns

1 bay leaf

2.5 litres (4½ pints) cold water

To serve

freshly chopped herbs

salt flakes

There is no need to discard the solidified fat you pick off. It can be frozen in small batches and added to dishes for extra richness and beefy flavour.

Preheat the oven to 220°C/200°C fan/425°F/gas mark 7.

Spread the bones out on a large baking tray and place in the oven for 20 minutes. Remove from the oven and add the chopped celery and onion to the tray, tossing them in the rendered fat from the bones to coat. Return the tray to the oven for another 20 minutes.

Tip the roasted bones, caramelized vegetables and all the tray juices into a large pressure cooker. Smash the garlic cloves with the back of a knife and add to the pressure cooker along with the black peppercorns and bay leaf. Top up with the measured cold water and bring to the boil. Skim off and discard any foamy impurities that rise to the surface.

Reduce the heat to medium and secure the lid of the pressure cooker. Cook for 2 hours.

Allow the pressure cooker to cool completely before safely decompressing. Use tongs to remove the bones and place them into a colander set over a bowl. Strain the broth through a sieve into a larger bowl, discarding the vegetables and all the other bits. Any broth or juice that runs off from the bones can also be added to the large bowl of strained broth. Place the bowl in the refrigerator overnight to allow the fat to settle and solidify on the surface. This makes it easier to pick off the fat (see Tip). You will be left with a clear, clarified, full-flavoured bone broth.

It will be gelatinous, so portion it as needed and reheat gently before enjoying with plenty of freshly chopped herbs and salt flakes.

Chicken Broth

This homemade broth reminds me of homemade chicken soup from my childhood. I roast the bones and carcasses of chicken (my butcher gives them to me at no cost), then cook them in a pressure cooker with some keto-friendly vegetables. I then chill the broth in the refrigerator overnight, making it easier to remove the fat that solidifies on the surface. I do this because I like a clear broth, but that step is entirely optional. This is a hearty, delicious and surprisingly filling little meal. *Pictured on page 3.*

 9–10 SERVINGS **10m** PREP TIME **3hrs** COOK TIME **12hrs** CHILLING TIME

1.6kg (3lb 8oz) raw chicken carcasses

10g (¼oz) lard

2 celery stalks, roughly chopped

1 large onion, roughly chopped

3 garlic cloves

½ teaspoon whole black peppercorns

1 bay leaf

2.5 litres (4½ pints) cold water

salt flakes, to serve

As with the Beef Bone Broth, there is no need to discard the fat you pick off. It can be reserved and added to casseroles, vegetables or sauces for additional flavour.

Preheat the oven to 220°C/200°C fan/425°F/gas mark 7.

Spread the carcasses out on a large baking tray and place in the oven for 40 minutes until they have turned golden. Remove and set aside.

Melt the lard in a pressure cooker over a high heat and fry the celery and onion until caramelized.

Add the roasted chicken pieces to the pressure cooker and tip in all the rendered fat and juices from the tray they were roasted in. Smash the garlic cloves with the back of a knife and add to the pressure cooker along with the black peppercorns and bay leaf. Top up with the measured cold water and bring to the boil. Skim off and discard any foamy impurities that rise to the surface.

Reduce the heat to medium and secure the lid of the pressure cooker. Cook for 2 hours.

Allow the pressure cooker to cool completely before safely decompressing. Strain the mixture through a fine mesh sieve into a larger bowl, discarding the vegetables and bones.

Place in the refrigerator overnight to allow the fat to settle on the surface. This makes it easier to pick off the fat (see Tip). You will be left with a clear, full-flavoured chicken broth. Portion as needed and reheat before enjoying – and don't forget to add salt to boost all that lovely flavour.

Creamy Cauliflower Mash

I dare you not to love this! I mash up cooked cauliflower, add full-fat cream cheese and blitz the mixture to a very smooth purée (a step that is optional but encouraged). It's an incredibly versatile side dish that has myriad uses. You can serve just about anything with it – especially those dishes that need something to mop up flavourful sauces. *Pictured on page 95.*

4 SERVINGS AS A SIDE | **10m** PREP TIME | **20m** COOK TIME

CALORIES 137 | CARBOHYDRATES 5.8G | PROTEIN 6.6G | FAT 9.1G

650g (1lb 7oz) cauliflower florets (approximately 1 very large head)

65g (2½oz) full-fat cream cheese

20g (¾oz) unsalted butter

salt and ground white pepper

Trim the cauliflower into equal-sized pieces while you bring a pan of salted water to the boil. Add the florets to the boiling water and cook until they have softened completely – this can take up to 20 minutes. To test, pierce a floret with a fork – it should slide off instantly.

Drain the cooked cauliflower in a colander and leave to steam off for a few minutes (this important step will ensure you don't have a watery mash).

Transfer the mixture to a large bowl (or simply return it to the same pan, wiped dry with kitchen paper) and use a potato masher to mash well. Add the cream cheese and season generously with salt and white pepper.

Tip the mash into a food processor and blitz until smooth. Taste and adjust the seasoning with more salt and pepper if needed, then stir in the butter just before serving.

Garlic Butter Cauliflower Rice

This method of cooking a cauliflower 'rice' delivers a fantastic texture and flavour and it beats all the other methods I have played around with. Don't blitz the cauliflower too finely as this will make it more likely to burn. *Pictured on pages 67 and 77.*

4 SERVINGS AS A SIDE | **15m** PREP TIME | **25m** COOK TIME

CALORIES 202 | CARBOHYDRATES 4.4G | PROTEIN 5G | FAT 18G

530g (1lb 3oz) cauliflower florets (approximately 1 large head)

50g (1¾oz) unsalted butter

1 teaspoon garlic powder

2 tablespoons olive oil

small handful flat-leaf parsley, finely chopped

salt and ground white pepper

Preheat the oven to 220°C/200°C fan/425°F/gas mark 7.

Blitz the cauliflower florets in a food processor until they resemble coarse breadcrumbs (see note above). Transfer into a large bowl.

Melt the butter in a small pan over a high heat. Once it starts foaming, pour it over the cauliflower. Add the garlic powder, season with salt and white pepper and mix. Spread in an even layer in a large baking tray.

Place in the oven for 10 minutes, then remove and stir. This will ensure even cooking and prevent thinner-spread layers burning. Return to the oven for an additional 10–12 minutes.

Before serving, drizzle over the olive oil and stir through the parsley.

Buttered Courgetti

You can buy ready-made 'courgetti', but nothing beats the freshness of spiralizing fresh courgettes yourself using an inexpensive spiralizer. I love flash-frying these noodles in butter and salt, but you can play around with different herbs (see Tip.) *Pictured on pages 84–85.*

2 SERVINGS AS A SIDE | **15m** PREP TIME | **1m** COOK TIME

CALORIES 126 | CARBOHYDRATES 2.8G | PROTEIN 2.8G | FAT 11G

1–2 courgettes

25g (1oz) unsalted butter

salt

If you are serving this with Meatballs Marinara (page 93), why not fold through a little oregano? Or to serve with the Easy Thai Prawn Curry (page 57), try flash-frying the noodles in coconut oil.

Use your spiralizer to create 300g (10½oz) 'noodles'. You can try a few different blade settings to find your preferred thickness.

Melt the butter in a large pan or wok over a high heat. Once it starts foaming, tip in the courgette noodles and fry for just 30–40 seconds, stirring constantly to ensure all the noodles are coated in the butter. You want the courgette noodles to retain some firmness, so be mindful of not overcooking them. The longer they cook, the more moisture will be released, and they will start to cook down and lose their shape and noodle-ness.

Season generously with salt and enjoy with your favourite saucy dishes!

Microwave Mug Breads

2
MUG
BREADS

5m
PREP
TIME

90s
COOK
TIME

White Mug Bread

50g (1¾oz) almond flour

1 teaspoon baking powder

½ teaspoon mustard powder

generous pinch of salt

2 large eggs

20g (¾oz) unsalted butter, gently melted

I often whip up a mug bread when the craving for a bacon sandwich strikes. Once you get the hang of it, you can enjoy them as you would any slice of bread (smashed avo, anyone?). I use the white bread version in the Mini French Toast Rounds (page 32) and the chia version is used in the decadent Salmon Eggs Benedict breakfast (page 26). I make both versions in ramekins, but suitably shaped, microwave-friendly mugs will work just as well. Simply put, you are 90 seconds away from a game changer! Both versions make two mug breads.

PER WHITE MUG BREAD | CALORIES 320 | CARBOHYDRATES 2.3G | PROTEIN 13G | FAT 28G

PER CHIA MUG BREAD | CALORIES 323 | CARBOHYDRATES 2.8G | PROTEIN 13G | FAT 27G

Both recipes follow the same method.

Simply combine all the dry ingredients very well in a bowl.

In a separate bowl, whisk the eggs very well before whisking in the melted butter. Pour the egg mixture into the dry ingredients and gently fold through to combine.

Divide the mixture between two greased ramekins or mugs and place them (one at a time) in the microwave on high for 90 seconds (see Tip).

Carefully remove from the microwave and slide a knife around the edges. Turn the ramekin or mug upside down to tip out the bread. Once cool enough to handle, turn each little 'bun' on its side and slice in half.

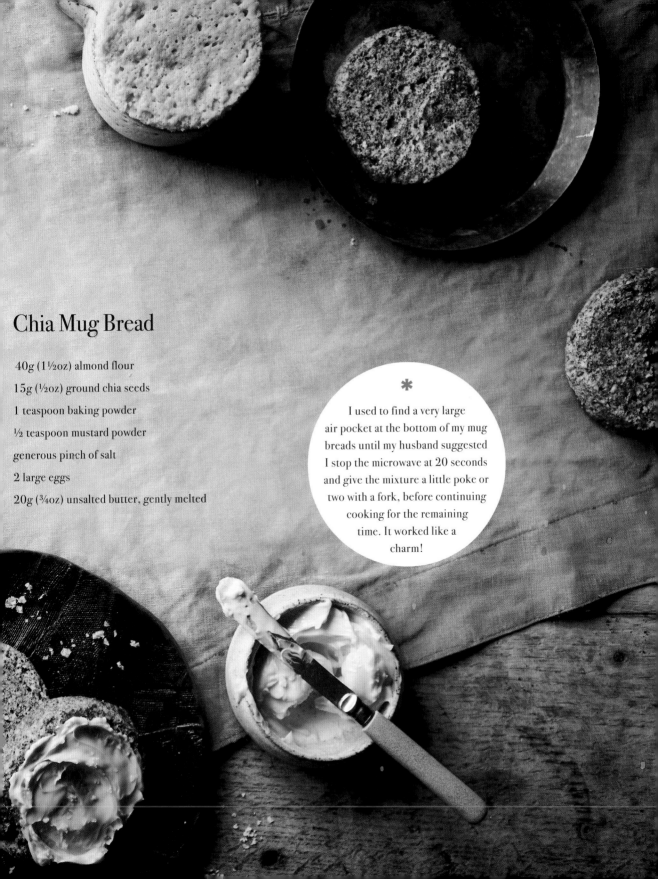

Chia Mug Bread

40g (1½oz) almond flour

15g (½oz) ground chia seeds

1 teaspoon baking powder

½ teaspoon mustard powder

generous pinch of salt

2 large eggs

20g (¾oz) unsalted butter, gently melted

*

I used to find a very large air pocket at the bottom of my mug breads until my husband suggested I stop the microwave at 20 seconds and give the mixture a little poke or two with a fork, before continuing cooking for the remaining time. It worked like a charm!

Mixed Seed Bread Loaf

1 LOAF

15m PREP TIME

50m COOK TIME

Don't be intimidated by the ingredients in this recipe. They are all easily available online or at most health food stores and you can find a carton of egg whites in the dairy aisle of most supermarkets. (Alternatively, you could simply weigh out actual egg whites, but then you may need some inventive ways of using all those yolks! I tested this, it takes about 12–13 eggs and is not worth the effort in my opinion.) This bread freezes well – slice it first, then freeze the wrapped slices. *Pictured on pages 12 and 107.*

PER SLICE (APPROX. 85G/3oz) | CALORIES 415 | CARBOHYDRATES 5.3G | PROTEIN 15G | FAT 35G

For the dry mix

415g (14½oz) almond flour

45g (1¾oz) ground chia seeds

45g (1¾oz) ground flaxseed

30g (1oz) sesame seeds

2 tablespoons psyllium husk powder

2 tablespoons baking powder

1½ teaspoons salt

For the wet mix

495ml (18fl oz) egg whites

75g (2¾oz) unflavoured coconut oil, melted

60ml (4 tablespoons) double cream

To finish

1 tablespoon sunflower seeds

1 teaspoon sesame seeds

¼ teaspoon poppy seeds

Failing to cool the loaf before slicing will result in crumbly bread, so restrain yourself! If any seeds fall off when slicing, scoop them up and pop them into your sandwich for flavour and crunch.

Preheat the oven to 230°C/210°C fan/450°F/gas mark 8.

Grease and line a medium (900g/2lb) loaf tin with parchment paper, ensuring there is some overlap at the sides of the tin. You can also find liners made exactly for this tin size – use whichever is more convenient for you.

Have two large bowls ready. In one, add all the dry ingredients and use a clean, dry whisk to combine well. In the second bowl, whisk together the wet ingredients (being sure that the melted coconut oil isn't too hot, as this may cook parts of the egg).

Tip the wet mix into the dry mix and use a wooden spoon to combine. Pour the thick mixture into the prepared loaf tin and gently smooth over. Scatter over the sunflower, sesame and poppy seeds and very gently press them into the surface.

Bake in the oven for 10 minutes, then reduce the temperature to 180°C/160°C fan/350°F/gas mark 4 (without opening the oven door) and continue to bake for 40 minutes.

Remove and place on a cooling rack for several minutes before lifting the bread from the tin and peeling away the parchment. Allow to cool completely before slicing (see Tip).

Soft Dinner Rolls

I have binned my fair share of duds over the years while developing keto bread. However, I have made this recipe often enough to know the results are consistently brilliant! Please stick to the recipe below for the best results. Omitting or replacing ingredients will lead to undesirable changes in texture and may even make the mixture unworkable. I must stress that your digital scale is vital in baking; weigh out exactly the amounts indicated to achieve the beautifully soft texture of these amazing little rolls. *Pictured on pages 8 and 55.*

9 DINNER ROLLS | **15m** PREP TIME | **30m** COOK TIME

PER ROLL | CALORIES 161 | CARBOHYDRATES 4G | PROTEIN 5.2G | FAT 13G

For the wet mix

60g (2¼oz) unsalted butter

4 large eggs

1 tablespoon olive oil

60ml (4 tablespoons) lukewarm water

For the dry mix

40g (1½oz) almond flour

40g (1½oz) coconut flour

25g (1oz) psyllium husk powder

1 teaspoon mustard powder

1 teaspoon baking powder

1 teaspoon salt

½ teaspoon garlic powder

For the topping

1 teaspoon sesame seeds

½ teaspoon poppy seeds

Preheat the oven to 200°C/180°C fan/400°F/gas mark 6 and line a small baking tray with parchment paper.

For the wet mix, melt the butter in a small pan over a low heat. Remove from the heat and allow to cool slightly. Whisk the eggs and olive oil in a bowl. Add the lukewarm water, then whisk in the melted butter.

In a second, larger bowl, combine all the dry ingredients very well. Pour in the egg mixture and mix to combine. At this stage, the mixture will look like a very lumpy batter. This is normal. Leave to stand for a minute to allow the psyllium husk powder to thicken the mixture.

The batter will have thickened enough to make it easy to work with, but it contains a lot of fat so it will still be very soft. If the batter is still too soft to work with after a minute of standing, it's likely your brand of coconut flour is a little different to mine. Mix in 1 tablespoon each of almond and coconut flour to achieve a mixture that you can handle, but please bear in mind that the mixture should still be very, very soft. If not, you will not get soft dinner rolls.

Divide it into 9 equal-sized portions and form into soft balls (approximately 50–55g/1¾–2oz each). Place onto the prepared baking tray, allowing plenty of space between each roll.

Scatter over the sesame and poppy seeds and bake in the oven for 15 minutes. Without opening the oven door, reduce the temperature to 170°C/150°C fan/340°F/gas mark 3½ and bake for an additional 12–14 minutes.

Tear apart and enjoy!

Homemade Mayonnaise

 MAKES 165G (5¾oz)

 15m PREP TIME

A little elbow grease and you are less than 15 minutes away from a 'clean' mayonnaise – free from any nasties found in the store-bought variety. Perfect for sandwiches with leftover meat and my Mixed Seed Bread Loaf (page 20) or either of the Mug Breads (pages 18–19).

CALORIES 276 | CARBOHYDRATES 0G | PROTEIN 0.7G | FAT 30G

1 large egg yolk

2 teaspoons white wine vinegar

1 teaspoon Dijon mustard

150ml (5fl oz) light olive oil (or avocado oil)

salt

Finely grate the zest of a lemon into the mayonnaise for a sharp lemon mayonnaise. Alternatively, you could add in roasted garlic or stir through finely chopped herbs of your choice.

Put the egg yolk, vinegar and mustard in a small jug and use a small whisk to thoroughly combine. (Placing the jug on a worktop lined with wet kitchen paper will prevent the jug from moving as you whisk.)

Drizzle very small amounts of the oil into the mixture at a time, whisking very well between each addition until emulsified. This must be done in stages to avoid the mixture splitting.

Once all the oil has been incorporated and the mixture has completely emulsified, you will be left with a thick, creamy, smooth mayonnaise.

Taste and adjust the seasoning with some salt. Cover and store for no longer than 4 days in the refrigerator.

Quick Salad Dressing

 ENOUGH TO DRESS A SALAD FOR 2–3

 5m PREP TIME

Store-bought dressings may be convenient, but they usually contain hidden sugars. Making your own dressing is fast and you can get creative with flavours. Just remember the simple ratio: one part acid (i.e. vinegar or lemon juice) to three parts oil. Go wild!

CALORIES 177 | CARBOHYDRATES 0G | PROTEIN 0.5G | FAT 19G

1 tablespoon white wine vinegar

3 tablespoons extra-virgin olive oil

1 teaspoon Dijon mustard

salt and freshly ground black pepper

Simply whisk together all the ingredients in a little bowl. If left to stand too long, the dressing may separate, although the mustard should do a good job of stabilizing the mixture. If it does separate, simply give it another whisk before dressing your salad.

Variations
– Use red wine vinegar or balsamic vinegar instead of white wine vinegar
– Use light olive oil or avocado oil for a lighter flavour
– Add a pinch of your favourite herbs (dried or fresh)
– Add crushed garlic or finely grated Parmesan for maximum punch
– Add finely grated lemon zest for extra zing

Roasted Tomato Marinara Sauce

MAKES 600G (1LB 5oz) | 15m PREP TIME | 1hr COOK TIME

This is a great sauce to master if you are steering clear of store-bought sauces that contain hidden sugars. I use this sauce in so many recipes, from Meatballs Marinara (page 83) to my keto pizzas (pages 47 and 92). For best results, use ripe, organic tomatoes on the vine.

PER 100G (3½oz) | CALORIES 76 | CARBOHYDRATES 5.4G | PROTEIN 1.1G | FAT 4.4G

4 large garlic cloves, unpeeled

2 tablespoons olive oil

1kg (2lb 4oz) ripe tomatoes, halved

1 tablespoon red wine vinegar

1 teaspoon dried oregano

1 teaspoon powdered erythritol

generous pinch of celery salt

generous pinch of dried thyme

salt and ground white pepper

Preheat the oven to 180°C/160°C fan/350°F/gas mark 4. Place the garlic cloves on a small sheet of kitchen foil. Drizzle over a tiny amount of the olive oil and wrap up into an airtight little parcel.

Place the tomatoes in a large bowl. Drizzle over the remaining olive oil and toss well to coat. Spread them (cut-side up) onto a large, greased baking tray, along with the foil parcel of garlic. Roast for 1 hour.

Scrape the roasted tomatoes into a bowl. Unwrap the garlic cloves, snip off the ends and squeeze the roasted flesh into the tomatoes. Add the red wine vinegar and blitz with a hand-held blender to your preferred texture. Stir in the oregano, erythritol, celery salt and thyme. Taste and season. Portion as needed, as this sauce freezes well.

Best-ever Homemade Pesto

MAKES 170G (6oz) | 20m PREP TIME

Homemade pesto doesn't last very long in our home due to its versatility and dynamite flavour. I love to use it in my Mozzarella Pesto Salad (page 48), Pesto-stuffed Chicken Breasts (page 73) and Monnie's Meatball Marinara (page 83). *Pictured on page 46.*

PER 40G (1½oz) | CALORIES 245 | CARBOHYDRATES 1.2G | PROTEIN 4.3G | FAT 25G

1 teaspoon unsalted butter

30g (1oz) pine nuts

3 garlic cloves, roughly chopped

30g (1oz) fresh basil leaves

10g (¼oz) fresh flat-leaf parsley leaves

30g (1oz) Parmesan, finely grated

70ml (2¼fl oz) olive oil

generous squeeze of fresh lemon juice

salt (if needed) and freshly ground black pepper

Melt the butter in a small pan over a low heat and lightly fry the pine nuts and garlic until golden. Remove the nuts and garlic from the pan and drain on a plate lined with kitchen paper.

Place the basil, parsley, grated Parmesan and olive oil in a mini food processor/food chopper. Tip in the pine nuts and garlic and add a generous squeeze of fresh lemon juice (catch the pips!).

Blitz well. Taste to check if it needs any salt seasoning (unlikely due to the Parmesan) and add a generous crack of black pepper.

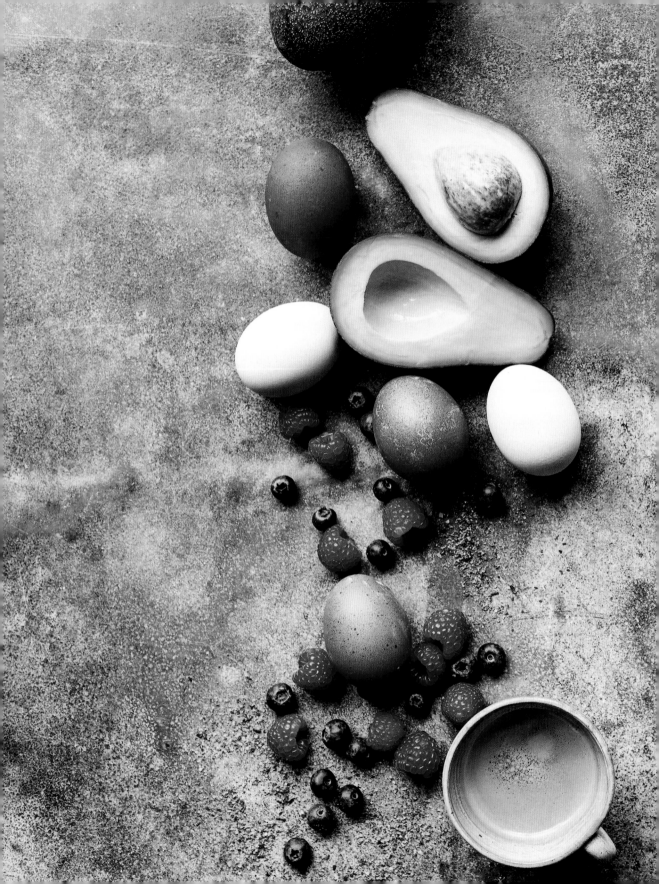

Breakfasts

Salmon Eggs Benedict

This is a mighty breakfast where each serving is exactly as pictured: two halves of toasted Chia Mug Bread (pages 18–19) topped with smoked salmon and perfectly poached eggs. The whole lot is then smothered in an easy keto Hollandaise sauce. It's the perfect option for weekend mornings when you wake up feeling creative and ambitious! At only 3.4g carbs per serving, you are safe in the hands of this rich brunch which will keep you satisfied well into the day!

 2 SERVINGS

 10m PREP TIME

 30m COOK TIME

CALORIES 906 | CARBOHYDRATES 3.4G | PROTEIN 50G | FAT 75G

2 Chia Mug Breads (pages 18–19)

2 teaspoons unsalted butter

1 tablespoon white vinegar

4 large eggs

160g (5¾oz) cold-smoked salmon

salt flakes and freshly ground black pepper

snipped chives, to serve

For the Hollandaise sauce

2 large egg yolks

1 teaspoon Chardonnay vinegar

50g (1¾oz) unsalted butter, softened

salt

Make the Hollandaise sauce by whisking the egg yolks and Chardonnay vinegar together in a heatproof bowl. At the same time, bring a pan of water to the boil. Position the bowl of egg yolks above the pan of simmering water and whisk continuously as you add the butter a little at a time.

Continue to whisk until all the butter has emulsified into the mixture. The sauce will thicken and become creamy. Season with salt and set aside until ready to use (you will notice it thickens further when standing).

Slice both mug breads in half, so you are left with 4 thick pieces. Melt the butter in a frying pan and cook the slices until toasted and crusty on both sides.

To poach the eggs, bring a pan of water to the boil and add the vinegar. Reduce the heat to a simmer and give the water a stir to create a swirl. Crack in the eggs, two at a time, and cook for 3–4 minutes before removing with a slotted spoon and placing onto a plate lined with kitchen paper.

Divide the salmon between the toasted bread slices. Place a poached egg on each slice and pour over the Hollandaise sauce. Season with salt flakes and freshly ground black pepper, then scatter over the snipped chives and serve.

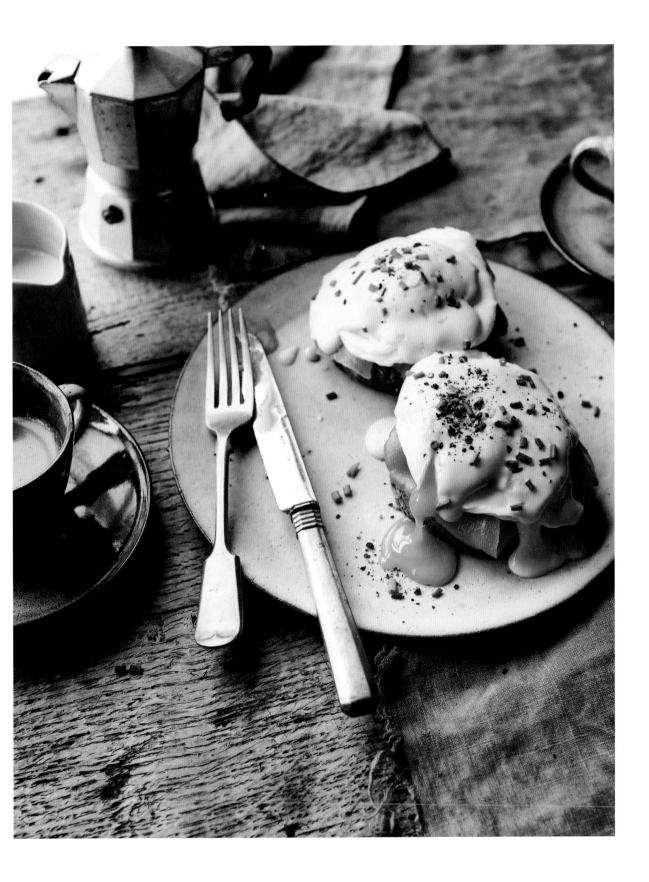

Cream-baked Eggs

If you need a little inspiration to jazz up eggs, may I remind you about the very simple classic dish of cream-baked eggs: uncomplicated, rich and packed with flavour. If you choose to add spice, try smoked paprika (which is excellent) or even ground turmeric. Ramekins are used in this recipe, but if you choose to use a wider, shallower dish, you may need to shave some time off the cooking. You can enjoy this scooped out, chopped up and served over a toasted Mug Bread (pages 18–19), but I simply dive into the ramekin with a teaspoon! *Pictured on page 31.*

CALORIES 351 | CARBOHYDRATES 0.7G | PROTEIN 16G | FAT 31G

2
SERVINGS

10m
PREP TIME

30m
COOK TIME

80ml (2¾fl oz) double cream

4 large eggs

generous pinch of salt flakes

pinch of ground white pepper

pinch of spice of your choice (optional; see recipe intro)

Preheat the oven to 200°C/180°C fan/400°F/gas mark 6 and have 2 greased ramekins ready.

Pour a little cream into each ramekin, then crack 2 eggs into each one.

Pour the remaining cream over the eggs and season with a generous pinch of salt flakes and a small pinch of ground white pepper. If you choose to add a spice of your choice, do so now. Very gently agitate the mixture with a teaspoon (I use my finger!) to spread the seasoning, but do not break the yolks while doing so.

Place the ramekins onto a baking tray (for easier removal) and bake for 25–30 minutes. Both the whites and yolks will set; this is normal.

Allow to cool for a minute before tucking in and please remember the ramekins are very hot!

Browned Butter Scramblies

Let's take scrambled eggs up a notch! Here, I quickly brown butter in which to cook the eggs and the resulting flavour is nutty and luxurious. I even add additional egg yolks for extra richness and colour – and you will love the subtle sweetness the flash-fried spring onions bring. This is a filling meal for any time of day. *Pictured on page 30.*

2 SERVINGS | **5m** PREP TIME | **5m** COOK TIME

CALORIES 304 | CARBOHYDRATES 0.7G | PROTEIN 19G | FAT 24G

4 large eggs, plus 2 large egg yolks

4 thick spring onions

2 tablespoons unsalted butter

salt and ground white pepper

salt flakes, to serve (optional)

Whisk the eggs and egg yolks together in a little jug or bowl. Season with salt and white pepper.

Trim the spring onions by slicing the white parts into very thick pieces. Keep them separate from the green ends, which should be thinly sliced and kept aside for later.

Melt the butter in a non-stick pan over a high heat. It will bubble and foam but will soon stop sizzling and you will notice a lovely, nutty aroma as the milk solids brown. Add the sliced white spring onions and fry them quickly until they turn bright green (this will happen in seconds).

Reduce the heat to very low and pour in the seasoned egg mixture. Stir continuously using a silicone spatula until just cooked through. This will take less than a minute; you want the eggs to be perfectly creamy without over-cooking them to a rubbery texture.

Serve immediately, topped with the green slices of spring onion and seasoned with salt flakes, if needed.

*

There is no need to discard the egg whites from the extra two eggs; they freeze well and can be used to make sugar-free meringues.

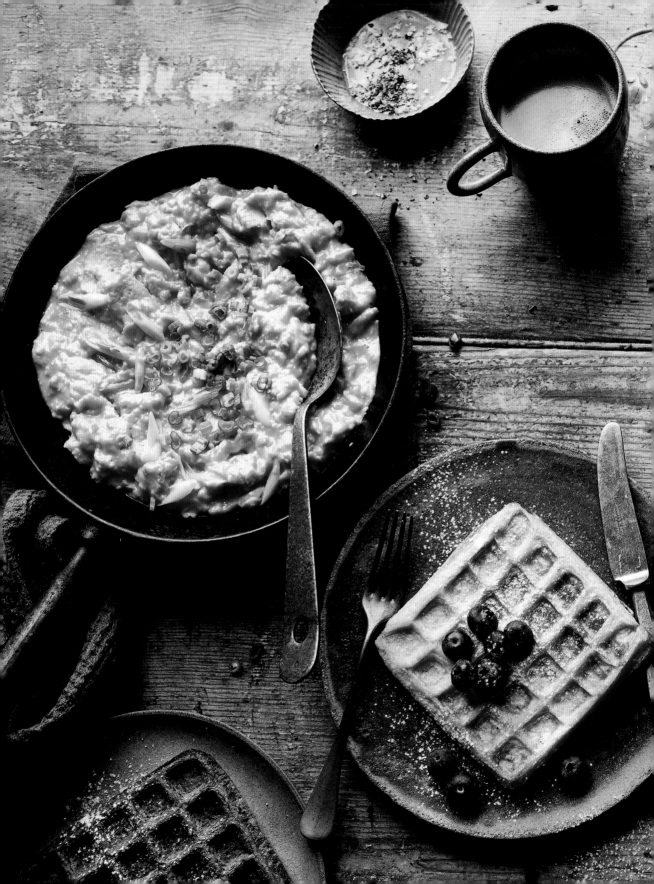

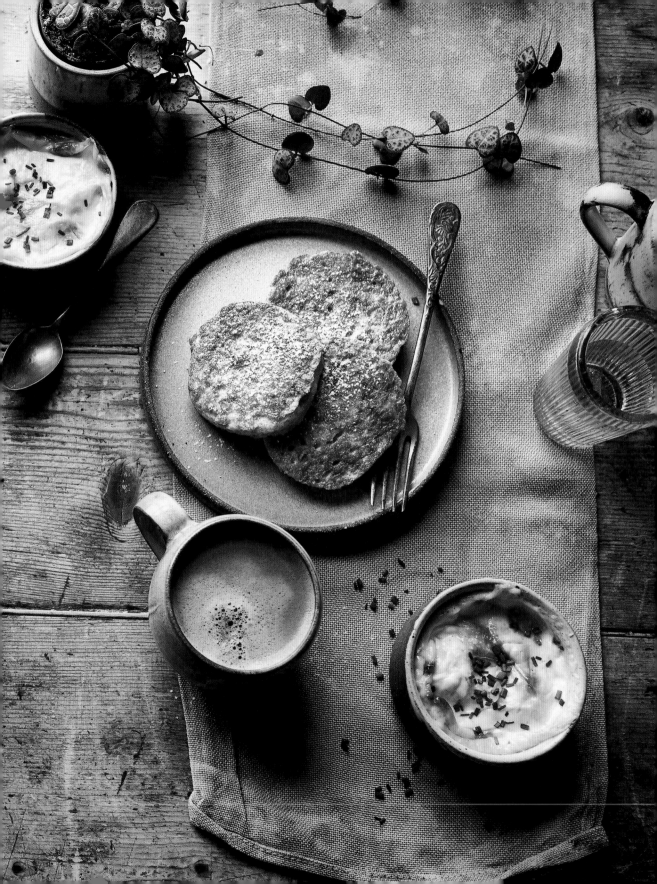

Mini French Toast Rounds

2 SERVINGS   **10m** PREP TIME   **10m** COOK TIME

2 White Mug Breads (page 18)

2 large eggs

20ml (¾fl oz) double cream

¼ teaspoon ground cinnamon

2 tablespoons unsalted butter

If you are making the sweet version, you could also dust over a little powdered erythritol before serving.

Yes, low-carb French toast is possible and happens to be very tasty, super quick and super easy! If you prefer your French toast savoury (like me), omit the ground cinnamon from the recipe below and season with a little salt instead. *Pictured on page 31.*

CALORIES 521 | CARBOHYDRATES 2.9G | PROTEIN 21G | FAT 46G

Slice each of the White Mug Breads into 3 thin slices so you are left with 6 mini rounds.

Whisk together the eggs, double cream and ground cinnamon in a bowl.

Melt the butter in a large, non-stick pan over a medium–high heat. Dip each of the bread rounds into the egg mixture and use your hands to compress them down to soak up the liquid. Lift and drain off any excess mixture, then add to the hot pan, frying until the rounds are golden on all sides. Remove and serve.

Keto 'Granola'

1 BATCH   **15m** PREP TIME   **10m** COOK TIME

50g (1¾oz) mixed seeds

70g (2½oz) raw unsalted mixed nuts, roughly chopped

10g (¼oz) unsweetened coconut flakes

generous pinch of powdered erythritol

This sweet keto 'granola' makes a fantastic topping when a dish may benefit from extra flavour and texture – for example, the Raspberry Yogurt or Overnight Chia Pots (page 36). Mixed raw nuts are widely available; just be sure that peanuts are not included in the mix.

PER 1 TABLESPOON GRANOLA | CALORIES 76 | CARBOHYDRATES 1.3G | PROTEIN 2.2G | FAT 6.7G

Preheat the oven to 200°C/180°C fan/400°F/gas mark 6.

Line a large baking tray with parchment paper and spread out the mixed seeds and nuts on it. Bake for 8–10 minutes, shaking and rotating the tray halfway through. Stir in the coconut flakes and return the tray to the oven for just 1 more minute (the coconut flakes burn quickly).

Remove from the oven and immediately scatter over the erythritol. Toss well to coat, then set aside to cool completely. Once cooled, store in a sealed container. The granola will keep for up to 2 weeks.

Waffles!

2 SERVINGS | 10m PREP TIME | 10m COOK TIME

Crispy on the outside, fluffy on the inside, this recipe is an excellent reason to invest in a waffle maker! I have based the macros on this recipe serving two, but waffle makers vary in size, so adjust accordingly for your waffle maker. *Pictured on page 30.*

CALORIES 361 | CARBOHYDRATES 4.1G | PROTEIN 19G | FAT 29G

4 large eggs

110g (4oz) full-fat cream cheese

20g (¾oz) almond flour

3 tablespoons powdered erythritol, sifted

1 teaspoon baking powder

Add a tablespoon of cocoa powder for chocolate waffles, or for a savoury version omit the sweetener and use a flavoured cream cheese.

Grease and preheat your waffle maker according to the manufacturer's instructions.

In the meantime, whisk the eggs in a bowl. Add the remaining ingredients and whisk very well to combine. You want a very smooth batter with no lumps.

When the waffle maker is ready, pour in the batter and cook until done (your waffle maker will alert you to this). Remove from the waffle maker and enjoy with melted butter or powdered sweetener and/or cinnamon dusted over. If you occasionally indulge in one of the sugar-free 'syrups' on the market, you could drizzle a little over your waffle.

Avocado & Berry Smoothies

2 SERVINGS | 5m PREP TIME

Smoothies are way better than juices as they retain all that lovely, glorious fibre. For the ultimate breakfast, I added MCT oil and collagen powder (optional, but included in the nutritional breakdown). *Pictured on page 34.*

CALORIES 401 | CARBOHYDRATES 7.6G | PROTEIN 9.2G | FAT 34G

200g (7oz) chopped avocado

220g (7¾oz) raspberries

2 tablespoons powdered erythritol, sifted

500ml (18fl oz) ice-cold water

2–3 drops liquid stevia (optional)

2 tablespoons MCT oil (optional)

2 tablespoons collagen protein powder (optional)

Simply add all the ingredients to a blender and blitz until smooth. Serve chilled.

– MCT oil is a supplement made from fats that are Medium-Chain Triglycerides. A little added to your morning smoothie or coffee can be an excellent energy source and promote a feeling of fullness. Introduce it into your diet in small amounts at first to avoid any digestive discomfort.
– Collagen protein powder supports our joints, muscles, bone and gut health as we age. It can simply be added to smoothies, soups or casseroles.

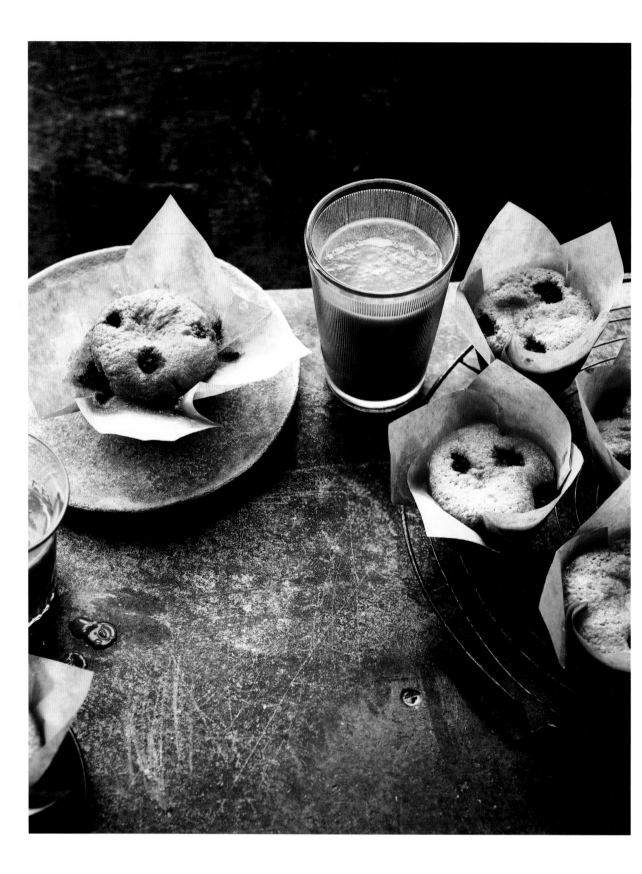

Blueberry Breakfast Muffins

It's only my husband and me in our home so I often share creations like this with our neighbours, who are also living low-carb. I do, however, keep a sneaky few muffins in the freezer because they are perfect for something sweet in the mornings. The macros are calculated using regular muffin cases, yielding 12 muffins, but if you choose to use tulip cases (as pictured) you could get away with using more filling in each. In that case, you will likely only yield about 10 muffins.

CALORIES 202 | CARBOHYDRATES 3.3G | PROTEIN 5.8G | FAT 18G

10-12 SERVINGS   **20m** PREP TIME   **30m** COOK TIME

80g (3oz) unflavoured coconut oil

4 large eggs

100g (3½oz) soured cream

4–5 drops liquid stevia (optional)

150g (5½oz) almond flour

30g (1oz) coconut flour

pinch of salt

1 teaspoon baking powder

1 teaspoon bicarbonate of soda

110g (4oz) powdered erythritol

100g (3½oz) small blueberries

If you do not want the tops to darken too much, gently lay a sheet of kitchen foil over the muffin tray after the first 10 minutes of baking, but do so quickly to avoid too much heat being lost while the oven door is open.

Preheat the oven to 180°C/160°C fan/350°F/gas mark 4. Line a muffin tin with 10–12 greased paper cases (see note in recipe intro).

Melt the coconut oil over a very low heat in a small pan. Remove from the heat and allow to cool slightly.

Crack the eggs into a bowl. Add the soured cream, melted coconut oil and liquid stevia (if using). Whisk well until you achieve a smooth, emulsified mixture.

In a second large bowl, combine the almond flour, coconut flour and salt. Sift in the baking powder, bicarbonate of soda and erythritol. Combine very well using a dry whisk to ensure the baking powder and bicarbonate of soda are evenly distributed.

Pour the wet egg mixture into the dry flour mixture and mix thoroughly to combine. Divide the batter evenly between the paper cases.

Top each muffin with an equal amount of blueberries. I don't bother mixing the blueberries into the batter, because gravity will do its thing when the muffins are in the oven.

Place the tray on the lowest rack and bake for 10 minutes (see Tip). Then reduce the temperature to 160°C/140°C fan/325°F/gas mark 3 and bake for an additional 15–18 minutes (or until a cake tester comes out clean when inserted).

Remove the cases from the muffin tray and set aside to cool on a cooling rack. These can be stored in the refrigerator or wrapped up individually and frozen. A quick defrost (a few hours at room temperature) and a couple of seconds in the microwave will breathe a little life into each one again.

Overnight Chia Pots

A few minutes of prep the night before is all it takes for this satisfying, high-fibre, grab-and-go breakfast option.

 2 SERVINGS   **5m** PREP TIME   **10m** COOK TIME   **12hrs** SETTING TIME

CALORIES 205 | CARBOHYDRATES 4.5G | PROTEIN 5.5G | FAT 17G

40g (1½oz) whole chia seeds

200ml (7fl oz) unsweetened almond milk

50g (1¾oz) blueberries

2 tablespoons powdered erythritol, sifted

2 tablespoons double cream

2–3 drops liquid stevia (optional)

Place the chia seeds in a bowl along with the almond milk. Cover and place in the refrigerator overnight for the seeds to soften and swell. After the first hour or two, give it a good stir to avoid any clumping.

Meanwhile, place the blueberries and a small splash of water in a small pan over a medium heat. After a minute or two, squash the blueberries with the back of a fork. Continue to stir and squash until you have a thick purée and all the water has evaporated. Set aside to cool, then cover and place in the refrigerator overnight.

The next morning, stir the erythritol, double cream and liquid stevia (if using) into the softened chia mixture, then fold in the blueberry purée. Divide between 2 serving pots before enjoying.

Raspberry Yogurt
with Flax & Keto 'Granola'

Here, I simply combine full-fat plain yogurt with whipped cream, then enhance the mixture with sweet raspberries. The ground flax adds fibre along with a lovely 'bran' flavour that reminds me of the milk I slurped up as a child after finishing a bowl of Bran Flakes.

 4 SERVINGS   **15m** PREP TIME   **10m** COOK TIME

CALORIES 227 | CARBOHYDRATES 4.7G | PROTEIN 7G | FAT 19G

100ml (3½fl oz) double cream

200g (7oz) full-fat plain yogurt

2 tablespoons ground flaxseed

1½ tablespoons powdered erythritol, sifted

2–3 drops liquid stevia (optional)

140g (5oz) raspberries, diced small

4 tablespoons Keto 'Granola' (page 32)

Start by whipping the cream to stiff peaks, then fold in the yogurt. Add the ground flaxseed, erythritol and liquid stevia (if using). Set aside until needed. This mixture can be made ahead of time.

You can either combine the yogurt cream with the diced raspberries and divide between 4 bowls, or if you are feeling fancy, you can layer the yogurt cream and raspberries. Just before serving, top each with a tablespoon of the keto 'granola' for delicious crunch.

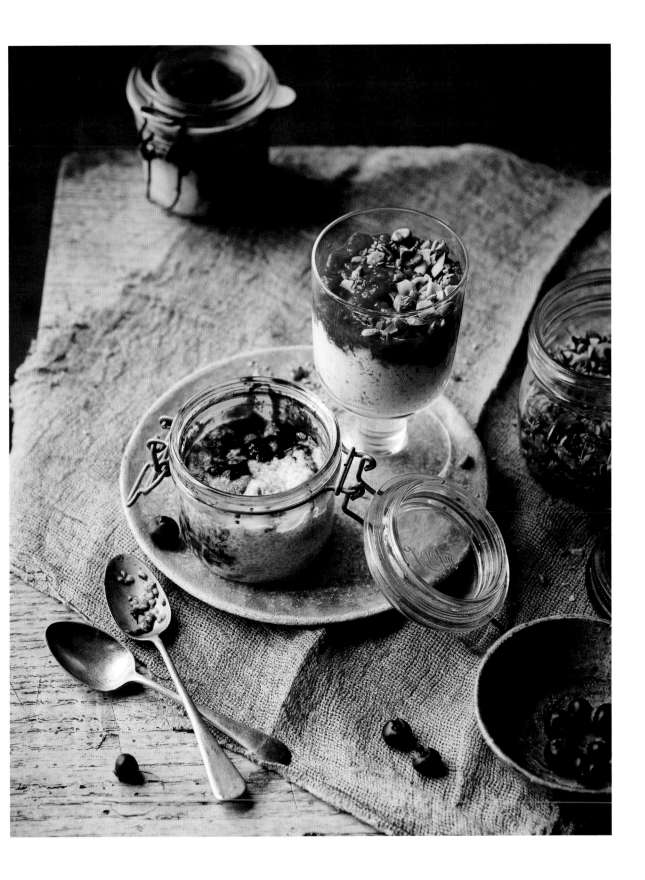

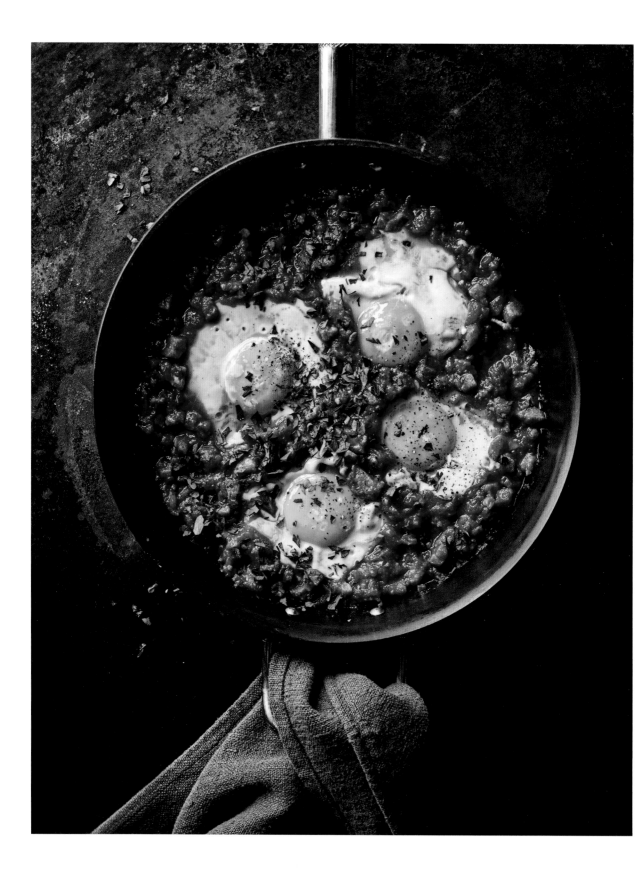

Shakshuka
with Smoky Pancetta

A spicy, smoky breakfast that makes for a hearty meal – suitable for any time of the day. Take the pan to the table as is and simply let your guests tuck in. The macros are calculated to serve two, but the dish can easily be stretched to serve four if accompanied by a slice or two of either of the Mug Bread recipes (pages 18–19). Also, remember that smoked pancetta lardons tend to be very salty, so season with salt (after cooking) only if you feel it's needed.

2 SERVINGS | **10m** PREP TIME | **30m** COOK TIME

CALORIES 373 | CARBOHYDRATES 4.2G | PROTEIN 27G | FAT 26G

130g (4¾oz) smoked pancetta lardons

250g (9oz) chopped tomatoes, canned or fresh

½ teaspoon ground cumin

¼ teaspoon smoked paprika

pinch of cayenne pepper

4 large eggs

salt (if needed) and freshly ground black pepper

small handful of fresh flat-leaf parsley, finely chopped, to serve

Heat a large non-stick pan over a medium–high heat and add the pancetta lardons, cooking for a minute or two until they have cooked through and rendered their fat and juices.

Add the chopped tomatoes, cumin, smoked paprika and cayenne pepper. Stir well and cover the pan with a lid. Reduce the heat to medium and cook for 10–12 minutes until the tomatoes have broken up and softened. Once the liquid has cooked out and evaporated (remove the lid for the last few minutes to ensure this), use a spatula to create four holes in the mixture. Crack an egg into each hole and cook until the egg whites are opaque. This can take up to 10–12 minutes, but you could speed things up by covering the pan with the lid.

Season the dish with plenty of freshly ground black pepper (and salt, if needed).

Scatter over the freshly chopped parsley and tuck in!

Bacon & Cheese 'Muffins'

9 SERVINGS

10m PREP TIME

25m COOK TIME

What a way to start the day! These fluffy muffins are incredibly rich and filling and one in the morning will keep you satisfied well into the day. If you choose to freeze them, simply defrost overnight in the refrigerator before popping in the microwave to bring them back to life. Do change up the fillings: add your favourite spices or herbs, or you can fry up diced mushrooms and spring onions in place of bacon. You could also use a stronger cheese, like Gruyère, to pack more punch.

CALORIES 168 | CARBOHYDRATES 0G | PROTEIN 11G | FAT 13G

2 teaspoons unsalted butter

240g (8½oz) smoked streaky bacon, chopped very small

6 large eggs

100ml (3½fl oz) unsweetened almond milk

1 teaspoon baking powder

70g (2½oz) extra-mature Cheddar cheese, finely grated

2 teaspoons snipped chives

ground white pepper

The smoked bacon adds plenty of saltiness, so the mixture may not require any additional salt seasoning.

Preheat the oven to 200°C/180°C fan/400°F/gas mark 6.

Line a muffin tray with 9 paper muffin cases.

Melt the butter in a non-stick pan and add the chopped bacon, frying gently until all the moisture is cooked out and the bacon is partially crispy. Set aside to cool slightly.

Combine the eggs and almond milk together in a large bowl and sift in the baking powder. Whisk well to combine, ensuring there are no powder lumps. Add the finely grated cheese, cooked bacon bits (along with any pan juices) and the snipped chives. Season the mixture with white pepper (see Tip, left).

Divide between the muffin cases (see Tip, right). I use a small measuring cup to scoop the mixture in as opposed to simply pouring it in. This ensures that the bacon and cheese are evenly distributed between the muffin cases.

Bake in the oven for 20 minutes, then remove the cases from the muffin tray to cool a little before enjoying!

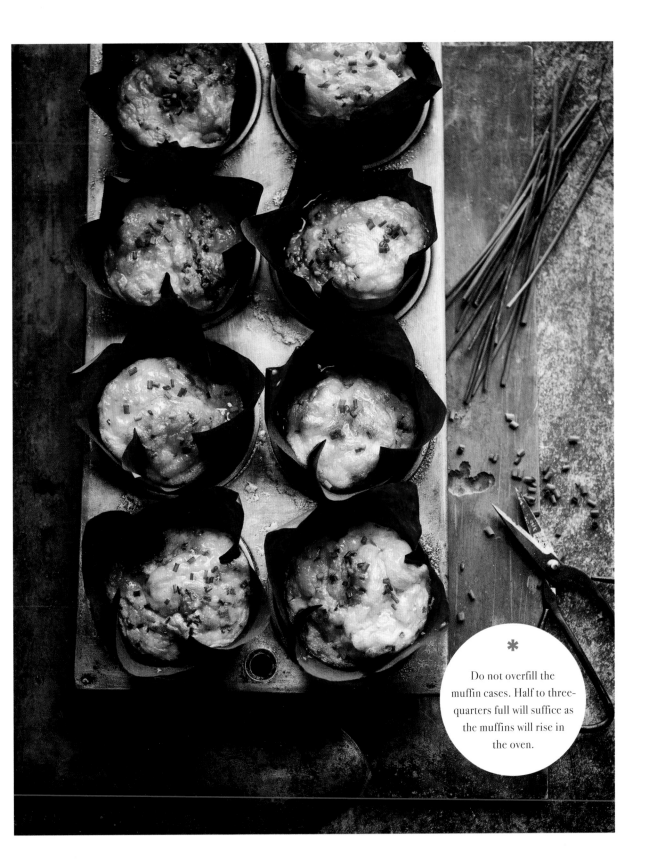

*

Do not overfill the muffin cases. Half to three-quarters full will suffice as the muffins will rise in the oven.

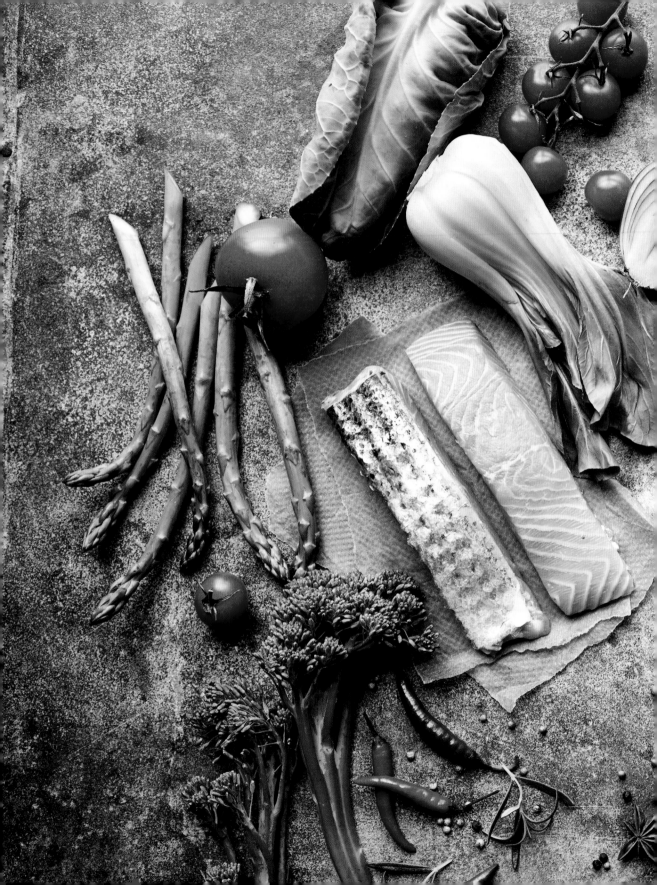

Keto
Meals

Crustless Tomato Quiche

I don't know what I did right (or wrong!) here, but this crustless quiche is the silkiest, creamiest one I have ever had. Sweet tomatoes are baked in a savoury custard and finished with mozzarella and (essential) basil. This is an easy meal to prepare and a great idea to take along to a picnic or pot luck. The quiche makes eight small slices and the macros are calculated per slice – so go on, have two!

8 SERVINGS | **10m** PREP TIME | **40m** COOK TIME

CALORIES 201 | CARBOHYDRATES 1.5G | PROTEIN 5.2G | FAT 19G

3 large eggs

180ml (6¼fl oz) double cream

75g (2¾oz) soured cream

75g (2¾oz) full-fat cream cheese

140g (5oz) cherry tomatoes, halved

55g (2oz) baby mozzarella balls, drained

salt, ground white pepper and freshly ground black pepper

small handful of fresh basil leaves, finely sliced, to serve

In case you didn't already know this, neither tomatoes nor basil should be stored in the refrigerator – they should be stored at room temperature.

Preheat the oven to 200°C/180°C fan/400°F/gas mark 6.

Grease a loose-bottomed 18cm (7in) tart tin and line the base with parchment paper. Place onto a baking tray.

Crack the eggs into a bowl and add the double cream, soured cream and cream cheese. Season with salt and white pepper, then use a whisk to mix well until completely smooth.

Pour the mixture into the prepared tin and add in three-quarters of the halved cherry tomatoes. Bake in the oven for 15 minutes.

Carefully remove from the oven and scatter over the mozzarella balls. Add the remaining tomato halves by gently lowering them into the partly cooked mixture. (This is for aesthetic purposes only, as the first batch of tomatoes will naturally sink).

Return to the oven for another 5–7 minutes, before turning the oven off. Leave the oven door slightly ajar and allow the quiche to finish cooking in the residual heat for about 10–15 minutes more. (It is normal for the very centre to look a little wobbly, but it should not be completely runny.)

Season with freshly ground black pepper and set on a cooling rack to cool. When ready to slice and serve, scatter over the freshly sliced basil leaves. The quiche can be enjoyed warm, cooled or at room temperature.

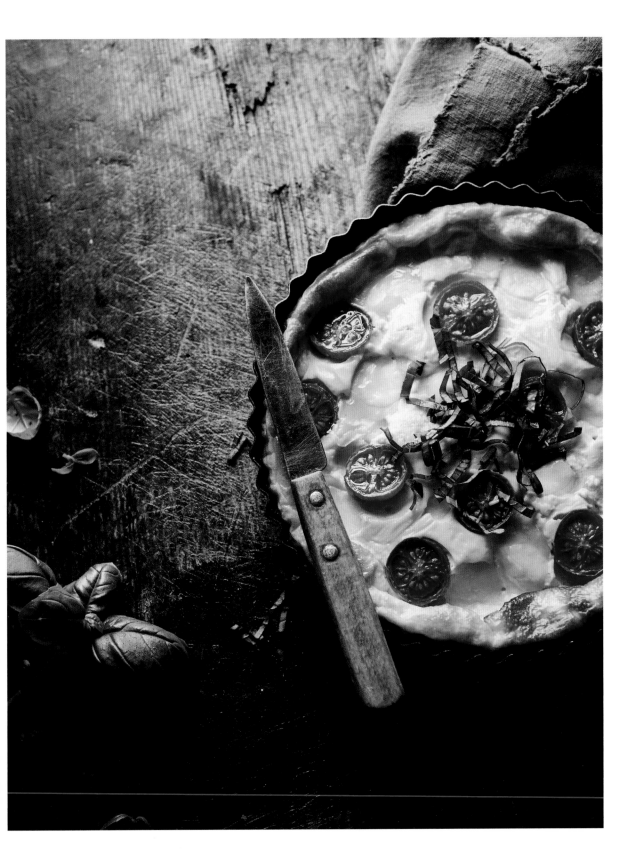

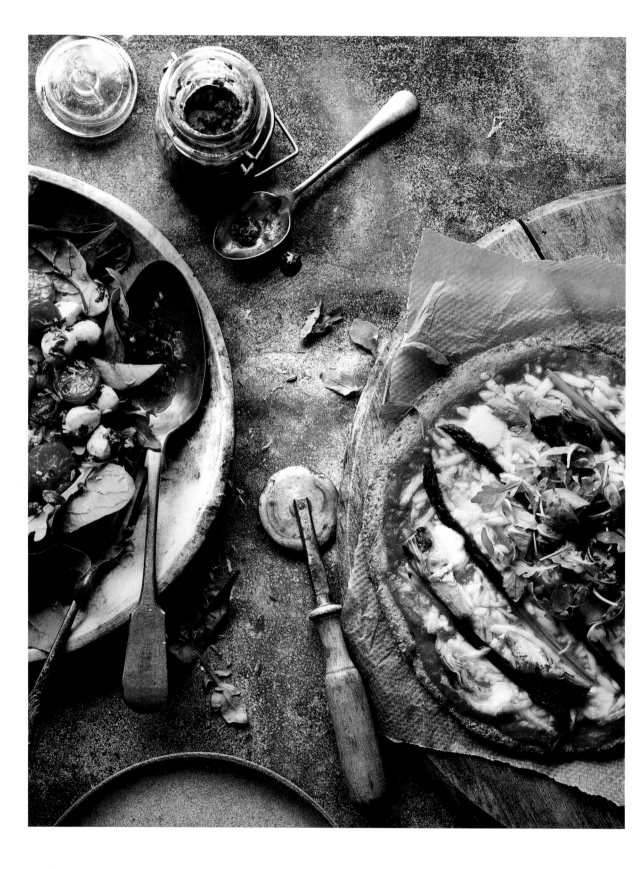

Cauliflower Crust Pizza

with Vegetables

2 SERVINGS

30m PREP TIME

30m COOK TIME

This is a lovely light pizza base option to try and is less heavy than the one featured on page 92. Sticking to vegetarian toppings, I used buttered fine asparagus and chargrilled artichokes (which you will find in the antipasti section in supermarkets). This recipe features my Roasted Tomato Marinara Sauce (page 23), so have that ready before you begin. Ready-grated mozzarella, while convenient, usually includes a small amount of potato starch. Try and source mozzarella you can grate yourself, or use fresh mozzarella torn into pieces.

PER ½ PIZZA | CALORIES 634 | CARBOHYDRATES 12G | PROTEIN 27G | FAT 51G

300g (10½oz) cauliflower florets

70g (2½oz) almond flour

1 teaspoon dried oregano, plus an extra pinch for sprinkling

1 teaspoon garlic powder

1 large egg, whisked well

1 tablespoon unflavoured coconut oil, melted

2 teaspoons unsalted butter

55g (2oz) fine asparagus

90g (3¼oz) Roasted Tomato Marinara Sauce (see page 23)

90g (3¼oz) grated pizza mozzarella

55g (2oz) chargrilled artichokes, drained on kitchen paper to remove excess oil

salt flakes and freshly ground black pepper

small handful of baby rocket leaves, to serve

Preheat the oven to 200°C/180°C fan/400°F/gas mark 6 and line a baking tray with parchment paper.

Blitz the cauliflower florets using a food processor. Place the blitzed cauliflower in a wide-bottomed bowl and cook on high heat in the microwave for 6 minutes. Tip the cauliflower into a colander lined with a large piece of muslin/cheesecloth. Once cool enough to handle, wrap the muslin/cheesecloth around the cauliflower and squeeze out all the liquid. This a very important step and will ensure a crust that you can pick up and eat like a pizza. If you do not remove enough moisture, your pizza base will be still be delicious, but much softer.

Empty out the cauliflower into a bowl. Add the almond flour, dried oregano, garlic powder, whisked egg and melted coconut oil. Mix well and season the mixture with salt and freshly ground black pepper.

Form the dough into a ball and place on the prepared tray. Use your hands to press down and shape the dough into a round shape of even height, to resemble a pizza base. Aim for approximately 5mm thick. Bake in the oven for 12 minutes, rotating the tray halfway through.

In the meantime, melt the butter in a pan over a low–medium heat and gently cook the asparagus for 1 minute. In a separate pan, heat the Roasted Tomato Marinara Sauce until it thickens.

After the 12 minutes have passed, remove the pizza base from the oven and spoon the tomato sauce evenly over it. Scatter over most of the grated mozzarella. Arrange the asparagus and artichokes on top and cover with the remaining mozzarella. Return the pizza to the oven for a further 10 minutes. Remove and sprinkle with a pinch of dried oregano and some salt flakes. Scatter over the baby rocket leaves and serve.

Mozzarella Pesto Salad

with Lemon & Fennel

This sensational salad combines powerfully flavoured Homemade Pesto (page 23) with fragrant, toasted fennel seeds and zingy lemon zest. These flavours work so well together, but I go a step further and semi-dry the cherry tomatoes to enhance their sweetness (a step that is optional, but encouraged). If you cannot source baby mozzarella balls (also called pearls), simply use regular buffalo mozzarella torn into pieces. To make this a more substantial meal, add grilled chicken pieces or boiled eggs. *Pictured on page 46.*

| 2 SERVINGS | 15m PREP TIME | 20m COOK TIME |

CALORIES 409 | CARBOHYDRATES 3.8G | PROTEIN 15G | FAT 36G

100g (3½oz) cherry tomatoes, halved

2 teaspoons fennel seeds

40g (1½oz) Homemade Pesto (see page 23)

125g (4½oz) baby mozzarella balls

finely grated zest of 1 lemon

2 tablespoons olive oil

2 large handfuls of mixed salad leaves

salt and freshly ground black pepper

Preheat the oven to 160°C/140°C fan/325°F/gas mark 3.

Spread the halved tomatoes out on a baking tray, cut side-up. Cook in the oven for 20 minutes to partially dry out. Remove and allow to cool.

In the meantime, toast the fennel seeds in a dry, non-stick pan until fragrant.

Combine the cooled tomatoes, toasted fennel seeds, pesto and mozzarella balls in a bowl, then add the lemon zest to the mixture. Season with salt and freshly ground black pepper, then stir in the olive oil.

You can leave this mixture to marinate until you are ready to toss it with your favourite salad leaves and serve.

*

Never dress salad leaves too far ahead of time – they will wilt and turn soggy. If you're taking this salad to work, keep the marinated mixture and salad leaves separate until you're ready to eat.

Smoked Salmon Salad

with Toasted Pine Nuts

This must be one of my favourite salads to throw together. Apart from the deliciously fatty salmon and avocado generously covered in fresh lemon juice, it boasts capers, toasted pine nuts and shaved Parmesan; that's just about all the ingredients I like best in one posh salad! If you decide to take this to work in a lunch box, I would advise only dressing the leaves with the oil and lemon juice just before eating to avoid them wilting. *Pictured on page 50.*

2 SERVINGS | **15m** PREP TIME

CALORIES 649 | CARBOHYDRATES 4.5G | PROTEIN 40G | FAT 51G

2 tablespoons pine nuts

1 generous handful of rocket leaves

1 generous handful of salad leaves

2 tablespoons olive oil

300g (10½oz) cold-smoked salmon

1 large avocado, peeled and diced

¼ red onion, thinly sliced

2 teaspoons capers, drained

generous squeeze of fresh lemon juice

salt and freshly ground black pepper

15g (½oz) Parmesan shavings, to serve

Toast the pine nuts in a dry pan over a medium heat until golden. Set aside to cool.

Combine the rocket and salad leaves and dress with the olive oil. Season with salt and freshly ground black pepper.

Add the smoked salmon, avocado, red onion and capers and generously squeeze over the lemon juice, along with another crack of black pepper.

Top with the toasted pine nuts and Parmesan before serving.

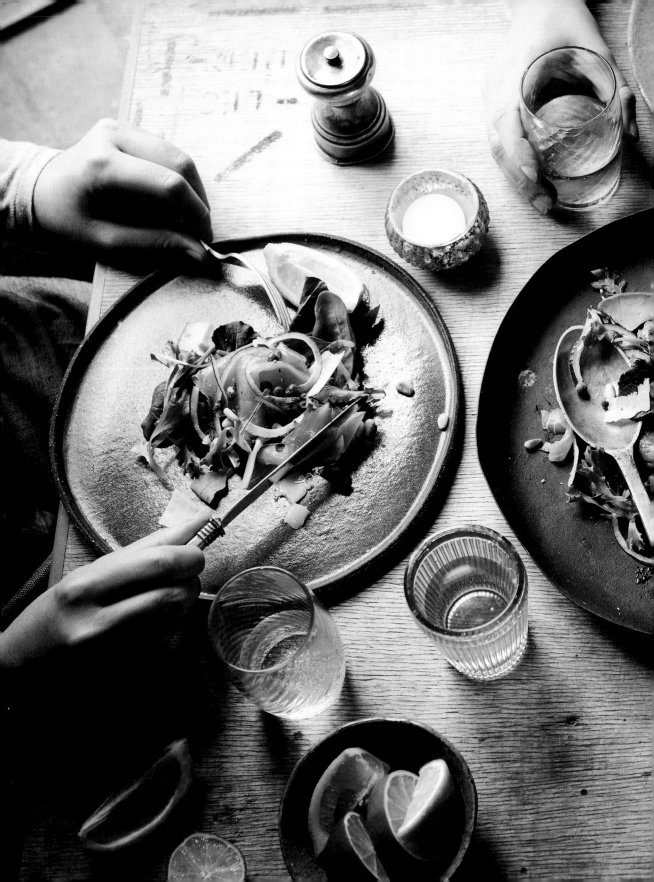

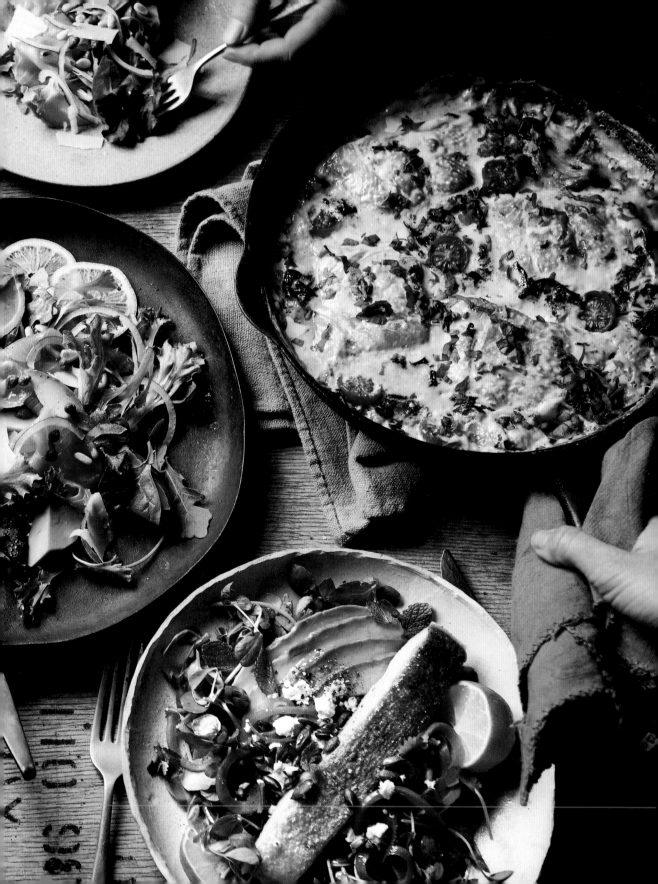

Salmon Salad

with Quick-pickled Onions

This spectacular salmon and avocado salad boasts a combination of flavours and textures that makes every mouthful perfect harmony! Small details, like toasting the pumpkin seeds beforehand, quick-pickling the thinly sliced red onions and using sesame oil create indescribable flavours. Simply put, you need to eat this! *Pictured on page 51.*

2 SERVINGS | **15m** PREP TIME | **20m** COOK TIME

CALORIES 670 | CARBOHYDRATES 5.1G | PROTEIN 38G | FAT 54G

½ small red onion, thinly sliced

1 tablespoon red wine vinegar

30g (1oz) pumpkin seeds

2 teaspoons unsalted butter

2 salmon fillets (approx. 130g/4½oz each)

1 lime, halved

handful of pea shoots

handful of watercress

small handful of fresh coriander leaves, finely chopped

small handful of fresh mint, finely chopped

1 tablespoon sesame oil (see Tip)

1 large avocado, peeled and sliced

30g (1oz) full-fat feta cheese, crumbled

*

If you can source toasted sesame oil (where production hasn't involved chemical solvents at high temperatures), this will maximize flavour in this dish.

Place the thinly sliced red onion in a little bowl and pour over the red wine vinegar. Toss to coat and set aside.

Toast the pumpkin seeds in a dry pan over a medium heat until they all pop open. Transfer to a plate and set aside to cool.

Using the same pan, melt the butter and cook the salmon skin side-down over a high heat for about 1 minute until the skin turns crispy. Turn each fillet and reduce the heat to medium, allowing the salmon to gently cook through for another 3–4 minutes. Squeeze one of the lime halves over the salmon and remove the pan from the heat.

Combine the pea shoots, watercress, coriander and mint in a bowl and squeeze the juice from the second lime half over the salad. Add the sesame oil and toss well to coat. Divide the salad between 2 bowls.

Drain the pickled red onions, discarding the vinegar. Serve the salmon and the sliced avocado with the salad and garnish with the red onions. Finish with a crumbling of feta and the toasted pumpkin seeds.

Creamy Salmon & Spinach Bake

This is my go-to dish when we entertain guests who love fish. It's an easy, simple and truly delicious one-pan dish. The acidity of the lemon squeezed over the dish at the end is essential, as is the parsley garnish, which offers a beautiful fresh top note. I love this over Creamy Cauliflower Mash (page 16) or Garlic Butter Cauliflower Rice (page 17) to mop up the dreamy sauce. *Pictured on page 51.*

4 SERVINGS | **10m** PREP TIME | **20m** COOK TIME

CALORIES 670 | CARBOHYDRATES 2.4G | PROTEIN 35G | FAT 58G

4 salmon fillets (approx. 130g/4½oz each)

1 tablespoon unsalted butter

2 garlic cloves, finely sliced

120g (4¼oz) baby spinach leaves

280ml (9½fl oz) double cream

100g (3½oz) cherry tomatoes, halved

juice of ½ lemon

salt flakes, salt and ground white pepper

small handful of finely chopped fresh flat-leaf parsley, to serve

Preheat the oven to 200°C/180°C fan/400°F/gas mark 6.

Pat the salmon fillets dry with kitchen paper and season with salt. Set aside.

Melt the butter in a large, ovenproof, non-stick pan over a low heat and gently fry the garlic until softened. Add the spinach and stir continuously until the leaves wilt. Pour in the cream to gently warm through and season with salt and white pepper.

Add the salmon fillets to the pan along with the halved cherry tomatoes. Bake in the oven for 15–18 minutes to allow the salmon to poach in the thick cream.

To serve, squeeze over the juice of half a lemon (catch the pips!) and season with salt flakes. Finish with a generous scattering of finely chopped parsley.

Curried Mussels

Cooking live mussels may sound intimidating, but you only need to do it once in your life to realize how simple it really is. The flavour possibilities are also endless; I love a simple garlic, white wine and parsley butter (who doesn't?), but I changed things up a bit here by making a quick curry. The nutritional breakdown is based on this recipe serving two, but if 11g carbs per serving doesn't fit well with your daily macros, you could stretch this between three or four people as an appetizer.

 2–4 SERVINGS   **30m** PREP TIME   **20m** COOK TIME

CALORIES 354 | CARBOHYDRATES 11G | PROTEIN 16G | FAT 26G

1kg (2lb 4oz) live mussels

2 teaspoons coconut oil

1 small celery stalk, very thinly sliced

3 garlic cloves, very thinly sliced

1 thumb-sized piece of ginger, peeled and minced

1 tablespoon medium curry powder

150g (5½oz) chopped tomatoes, canned or fresh

juice of 1 lime (plus extra if needed)

180ml (6¼fl oz) full-fat coconut milk

salt flakes

To serve

red chilli, very thinly sliced

handful of fresh coriander leaves

Never leave live mussels soaking in tap water – they will die. Keep the little guys in the refrigerator until cleaning them just before cooking.

Rinse the mussels well in a colander, picking off and discarding any beardy bits and grit. Selecting one mussel at a time, give it a little tap on your kitchen counter and watch closely; if it closes, it's alive and good to use. Set the good ones aside. If there are any that are completely closed, use them too; you can see after cooking if they were alive or not.

In the meantime, melt the coconut oil in a large pan (one that has a well-fitting lid) and cook the celery, garlic and ginger over a low heat for approximately 10–12 minutes until the celery and garlic completely soften. Add the curry powder and chopped tomatoes, stirring well until your mixture cooks to a non-watery purée.

Deglaze the pan with the lime juice, then throw the squeezed lime halves into the pan for additional flavour. Once all the liquid evaporates, pour in the coconut milk and increase the heat. Bring to a boil, stirring well and scraping down the sides of the pan. Allow the coconut milk to reduce by half.

Over a high heat, tip in all the mussels and cover with the lid. Cook for 90 seconds, picking up the pan to shake it once or twice during this time.

Serve topped with the sliced chilli and coriander leaves. Season with salt flakes and squeeze over additional lime juice, if needed. Discard any mussels that did not open after cooking.

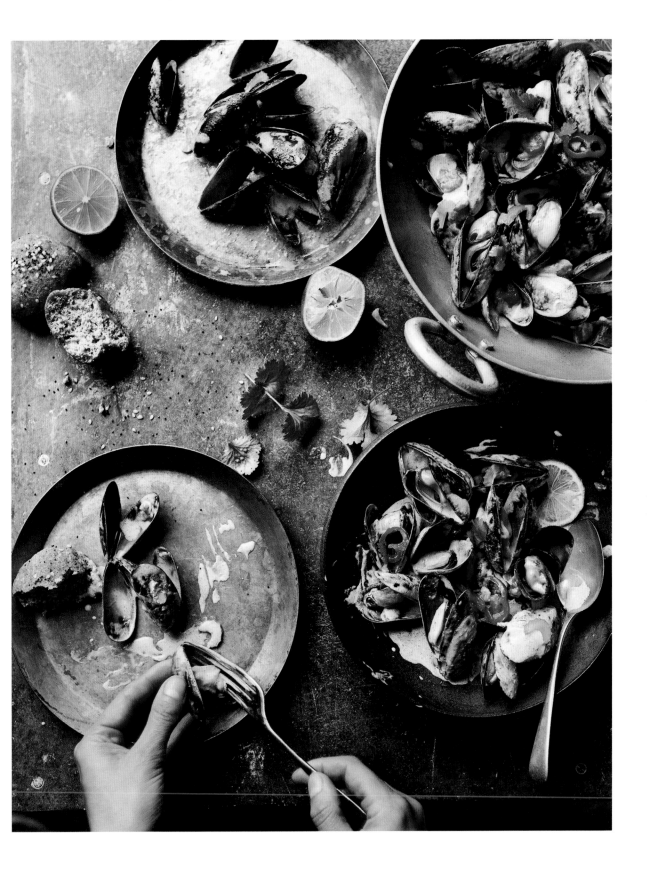

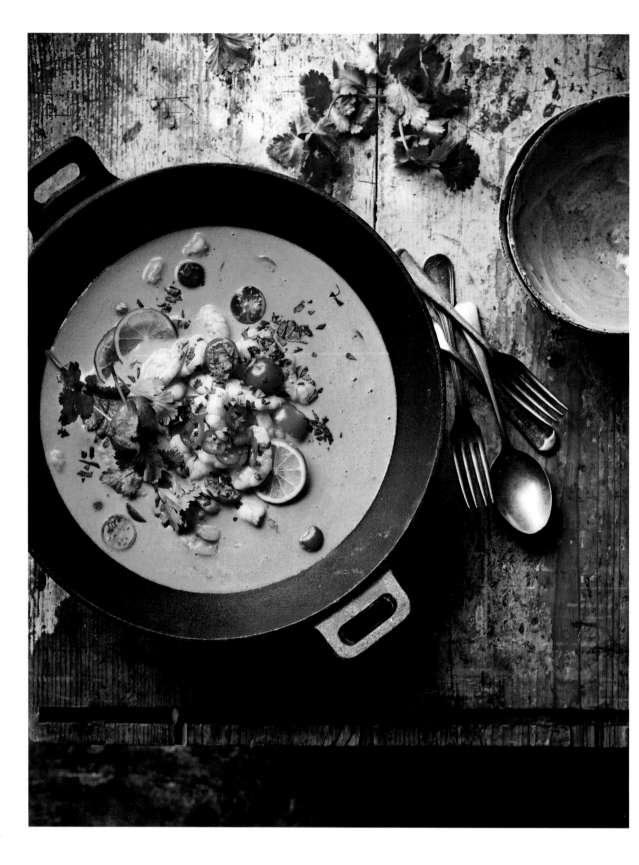

Easy Thai Prawn Curry

Fragrant, spicy, creamy ... this sensational prawn curry is made using a quick-and-easy homemade curry paste and coconut milk. The plump, perfectly cooked prawns, sweet cherry tomatoes, salty fish sauce, spicy chillies, acidic lime and fragrant coriander all create perfect harmony. I also added a little erythritol for some much-needed sweetness. Serve over Buttered Courgetti or Garlic Butter Cauliflower Rice (page 17) – or eat it straight from the wok, as I often do!

4 SERVINGS | **10m** PREP TIME | **30m** COOK TIME

CALORIES 387 | CARBOHYDRATES 8.3G | PROTEIN 24G | FAT 28G

For the Thai curry paste

2 large red chillies, deseeded and chopped

1 lemongrass stalk, roughly chopped (discard the hard outer layer)

½ red onion, chopped

4 garlic cloves, chopped

20g (¾oz) fresh ginger root, peeled and roughly chopped

½ teaspoon ground coriander

¼ teaspoon ground turmeric

pinch of ground cinnamon

2 tablespoons coconut oil, melted

For the prawn curry

1 tablespoon coconut oil

600g (1lb 5oz) uncooked king prawns, peeled

400ml (14fl oz) full-fat coconut milk

1 teaspoon powdered erythritol, sifted

1 teaspoon fish sauce

150g (5½oz) cherry tomatoes, halved

To serve

juice of ½ lime

handful of fresh coriander, finely chopped

1 red chilli, very thinly sliced

Make the Thai curry paste by simply adding all the ingredients to a mini food processor/food chopper. Blitz until completely smooth, stopping to scrape down the sides to ensure a very smooth mixture. Set aside.

For the prawn curry, heat the coconut oil in a wok over a high heat and flash-fry the prawns until they have turned pink. This doesn't take long and is best done in two or three batches to avoid overcrowding the pan. Remove the prawns from the wok and set aside.

Add the prepared paste to the same wok and cook for about a minute over a moderately high heat. Tip in the coconut milk and whisk well to combine, using a silicone-tipped whisk to avoid scratching your wok.

Stir continuously until the mixture reduces by at least three-quarters. This can take up to 15 minutes as you want the mixture reduced to a thick, creamy sauce.

Remove the wok from the heat and stir in the powdered erythritol and fish sauce. Return the cooked prawns to the wok and add the halved tomatoes. The residual heat of the sauce will warm the prawns through (without over-cooking them) and partially soften the tomatoes to perfection.

To serve, squeeze over fresh lime juice and scatter over the chopped coriander and red chilli slices.

Coconut 'Grits'

with Prawns & Bacon

Grits is a dish of Native American origin made using cornmeal. It is very popular in the southern states of America, but not very well-known in other parts of the world. Inspired by the concept, I created 'keto grits' by blitzing cauliflower florets, and threw in a few of my favourite ingredients to maximize flavour. This may look like a small meal, but don't be deceived – the rich flavour compensates!

2 SERVINGS   **15m** PREP TIME   **20m** COOK TIME

CALORIES 636 | CARBOHYDRATES 11G | PROTEIN 34G | FAT 49G

50g (1¾oz) desiccated coconut

1 tablespoon unsalted butter

250g (9oz) raw king prawns, peeled

100g (3½oz) smoked bacon lardons

2 garlic cloves, very thinly sliced

1 thumb-sized piece of fresh ginger, peeled and minced

3 spring onions, white parts thickly sliced, green ends thinly sliced and kept separate

120g (4¼oz) baby chestnut mushrooms, quartered

1 lemon, halved

170g (6¼oz) cauliflower florets, blitzed into 'rice'

170ml (6fl oz) full-fat coconut milk (see Tip)

salt

To serve

1 red chilli, thinly sliced

small handful of fresh coriander, chopped

Toast the desiccated coconut in a deep non-stick pan or wok over a medium heat. Stir continuously with a silicone spatula. Once golden, remove from the pan and set aside. It can burn quickly if you don't keep your eye on it.

Using the same wok, melt the butter over a high heat and flash-fry the prawns until they have turned pink and cooked through. Remove them using tongs or a slotted spoon, ensuring all the butter and juices remain in the pan. Season the prawns with a little salt and set aside on a plate to keep warm.

Tip the bacon lardons, garlic and ginger into the same wok and reduce the heat. Cook over a low heat until the bacon releases all its fat and juices and the garlic and ginger begin to soften. Add the spring onions (white parts only) and the mushrooms, cooking until the mushrooms have released their moisture and the pan starts looking dry.

Deglaze the pan with the juice of one of the lemon halves (catch the pips!) then add the blitzed cauliflower. Cook over a medium heat for 1–2 minutes, stirring continuously.

Pour in the coconut milk and most of the toasted desiccated coconut.

Cook for approximately 5 minutes over a low–medium heat until the coconut milk has reduced to a thick, creamy mixture.

To serve, divide the mixture between 2 small bowls. Top with (or stir through) the warm prawns and squeeze over the juice of the remaining lemon half.

Top with the remaining toasted coconut, the sliced green parts of the spring onions, and the red chilli and coriander.

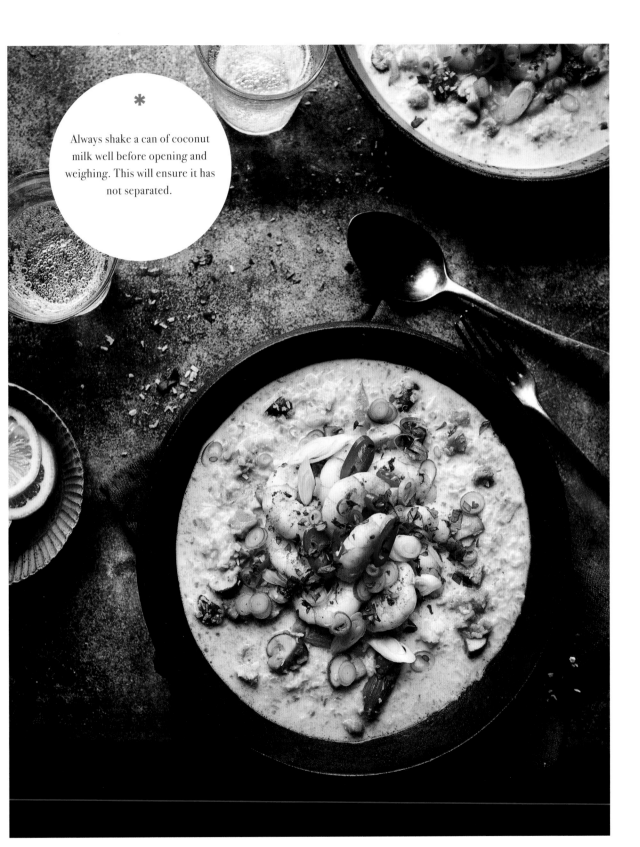

Always shake a can of coconut milk well before opening and weighing. This will ensure it has not separated.

Creamy Cod

with Jammy Onions & Dill

This tasty fish dinner boasts amazing flavours! I love the intoxicating flavour of baked cream but the real star of the show here is the jammy onion layer tucked under each fillet. The freshly chopped dill scattered over after baking is an essential top-note flavour that brings all the elements together. This is truly one of my favourite recipes in this book and I hope you love it as much as I do!

4 SERVINGS

10m PREP TIME

1hr COOK TIME

CALORIES 512 | CARBOHYDRATES 4.8G | PROTEIN 26G | FAT 43G

1 tablespoon unsalted butter

2 medium onions, very thinly sliced

2 teaspoons white wine vinegar

300ml (10fl oz) double cream

4 skinless cod fillets (approx. 140g/5oz each)

salt and ground white pepper

To serve

salt flakes

generous handful of fresh dill, finely chopped

Melt the butter in a small pan and add the onions. Cook over a low heat, stirring occasionally, until they soften and begin to caramelize. This can take up to 20 minutes. Add the white wine vinegar and continue to cook for an additional 5–10 minutes until the onions become dark and jammy. In total, the onions should be on the heat for about 25–30 minutes. It's worth the wait!

In the meantime, preheat the oven to 200°C/180°C fan/400°F/gas mark 6.

Grease a small, suitably sized baking dish that will allow your cod fillets to fit snugly together and spread the jammy onions out in it.

Place the cream in the same pan you used to cook the onions (why dirty another pan?) and season with salt and white pepper as you gently warm it through over a low heat.

Season the cod fillets with salt and white pepper and place them on top of the jammy onions in the baking dish. Pour over the warm, seasoned cream and bake in the oven for 20–22 minutes.

To serve, season with salt flakes and scatter over a generous amount of the all-important chopped dill.

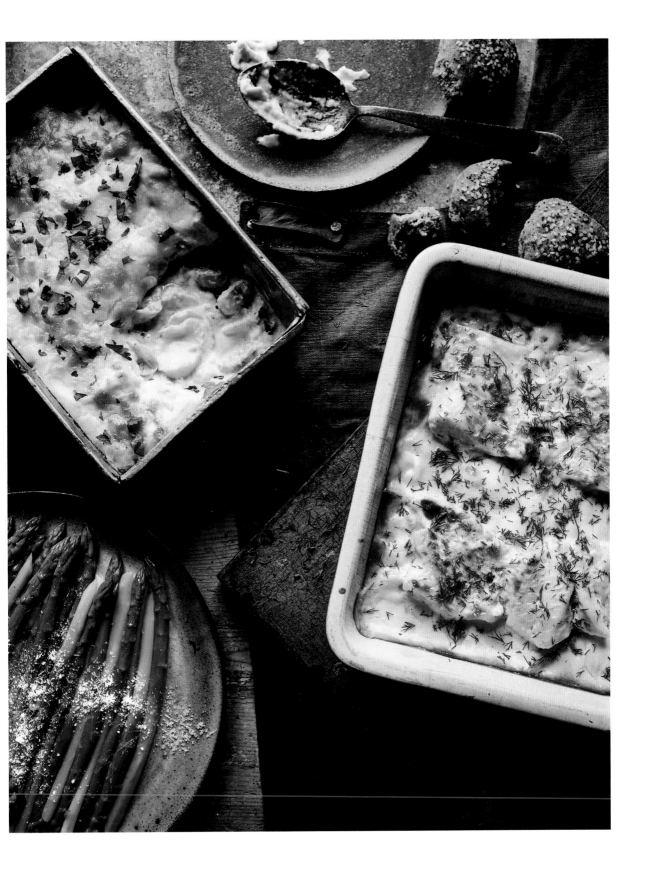

Comforting Seafood Pie

This is truly comfort food for seafood lovers! It's a generous, filling, hearty meal that the whole family will love. If you cannot source 'fish pie mix' (which most shops in the UK have conveniently put together for us), simply use equal amounts of skinned smoked haddock, white fish and salmon, chopped into small pieces. The smoked haddock is an important flavour element, so be sure it makes up a third of your fish. This recipe will yield four generous servings, but it's very rich and you will probably have leftovers. *Pictured on page 61.*

4 SERVINGS | **30m** PREP TIME | **1hr** COOK TIME

CALORIES 501 | CARBOHYDRATES 7.2G | PROTEIN 37G | FAT 35G

For the cauliflower mash topping

450g (1lb) cauliflower florets

45g (1½oz) full-fat cream cheese

2 teaspoons unsalted butter

salt and ground white pepper

For the fish pie

1 tablespoon unsalted butter

1 small onion, finely chopped

2 garlic cloves, crushed

50g (1¾oz) baby spinach leaves

juice of ½ lemon

2 teaspoons Dijon mustard

80ml (2¾fl oz) double cream

60g (2¼oz) soured cream

500g (1lb 2oz) fish pie mix (see recipe intro)

100g (3½oz) raw king prawns, peeled and halved lengthways

50g (1¾oz) extra-mature full-fat Cheddar cheese, grated

handful of fresh flat-leaf parsley, finely chopped, to serve

Preheat the oven to 200°C/180°C fan/400°F/gas mark 6.

Make the cauliflower mash topping following the method on page 16. Set aside to keep warm.

To make the fish pie, melt the butter in a large non-stick pan over a medium heat and cook the onions until completely softened. Add the garlic and baby spinach leaves and cook until the spinach wilts and releases all its moisture.

Deglaze the pan with the juice from half a lemon (catch the pips!) and cook until all the moisture has evaporated. Remove the pan from the heat and immediately stir in the mustard, double cream and soured cream. Tip in all the fish and prawns and stir well. Season with salt and white pepper, then tip the whole lot into a suitably sized baking dish.

Spread the cauliflower mash over the top and scatter over the grated cheese. Make a few small holes in the mixture using a chopstick or knife to allow excess steam to escape and minimize wateriness in your pie.

Place the dish onto a baking tray (this is for your own benefit, as the mixture is prone to bubbling over) and place in the oven for 25 minutes until the cheese is bubbling and the centre is piping hot.

Scatter over the chopped parsley just before serving.

Five-spice Duck Breast

with Pak Choi

Treat your loved one to this fancy-pants dinner, which takes just 45 minutes to throw together. Duck breasts are very generous in size and should be enjoyed pink on the inside with a crispy skin. Here, I use the flavours of fragrant Chinese five-spice to enhance the duck. I like to cook the accompanying pak choi until tender but still holding its shape. The whole dish is finished with an acidic drizzle incorporating all the fat and juices with some classic Asian garnishes. Just lovely! *Pictured on page 64.*

CALORIES 469 | CARBOHYDRATES 3.5G | PROTEIN 30G | FAT 36G

 2 SERVINGS

 15m PREP TIME

 30m COOK TIME

2 large deboned duck breasts (approx. 190g/6¾oz each)

1 teaspoon Chinese five-spice

2 pak choi, halved lengthways (larger ones may need to be quartered)

2 garlic cloves, thinly sliced

1 thumb-sized piece of ginger, peeled and thinly sliced

2 tablespoons rice wine vinegar

120ml (4fl oz) best-quality chicken stock

1 tablespoon unsalted butter

2 spring onions, thickly sliced

salt

To serve

1 red chilli, thinly sliced

small handful fresh coriander leaves

juice of 1 lime (optional)

Preheat the oven to 200°C/180°C fan/400°F/gas mark 6.

Remove the duck breasts from their packaging and pat dry with kitchen paper. Score the skin lightly and season both sides with a little salt.

Place the duck breasts skin side-down in a dry non-stick frying pan over a medium heat. Allow the duck skin to slowly render out its fat. After 15 minutes, you will notice a lot of rendered fat and juices. Increase the heat and cook until the skin is golden and crispy. (This method ensures a crispy skin that has not burnt.)

Flip the breasts over and cook the underside for 1 minute, spooning over the fat. Remove the duck breasts using tongs and place them, skin side-up, on a baking tray. Do not discard all the fat that remains in the frying pan.

Scatter most of the Chinese five-spice over the duck skin and use a silicone brush to brush a little rendered fat from the pan over the skins. Place in the oven for 6–7 minutes, after which you can remove the duck breasts from the tray and set aside to rest and keep warm. Do not turn the oven off. Pour out all the tray juices into a little bowl, as you will use later it in your sauce.

❋ *continued overleaf*

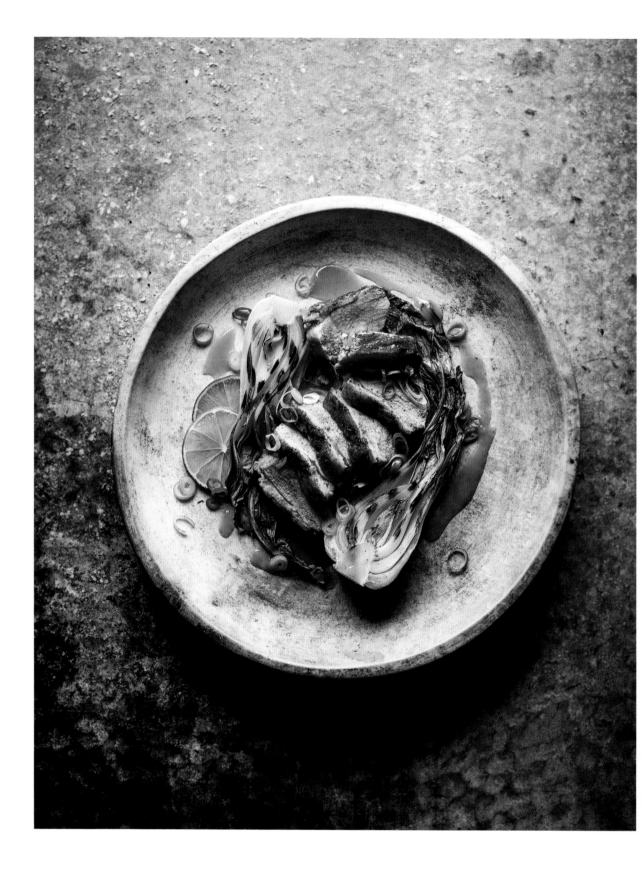

Five-spice Duck Breast

with Pak Choi
(continued)

In the meantime, use the same pan you fried the duck in to fry the pak choi over a medium–high heat until they get a little colour. There should be plenty of fat still in the pan to do so. Try and avoid burning the soft, green leaves. (I let the leafy parts overlap in the pan so that only the thick white section comes into direct contact with the hot pan.) Once browned, remove from the pan (again, leaving all the fat and juices in the pan) and place them on the same baking tray you used earlier for the duck. Place in the hot oven for 15 minutes to finish cooking through.

Add the garlic and ginger to the same frying pan you have been using all along (it should still have plenty of rendered fat and juices) and cook over a medium heat until the garlic begins to colour. Add the vinegar, chicken stock and the juices you reserved from finishing the duck in the oven. Add the remaining five-spice powder and cook this mixture for 5 minutes. Strain into a small, clean pan (discarding the ginger and garlic), then whisk in the butter until you have a thick, emulsified sauce. If it needs to thicken further, simply keep it on the heat longer until it has reduced sufficiently. Remove the pan from the heat and add the spring onions to gently warm through.

After the duck has rested, slice as you please and serve with the pak choi. Drizzle over the sauce and spring onions and top with sliced chilli and coriander. A squeeze of lime juice will finish it perfectly.

Lemon & Thyme Chicken

Deliciously zingy and packed with flavour, this is a simple dish that requires minimal effort and cleaning up. Frying the large chicken thighs skin side-down crisps the skin before they are baked, skin side-up, in a lemon, garlic and thyme chicken stock. The reduced cooking juices are then strained and further reduced to a thick glaze that is simply brushed over before serving. I love it served with Garlic Butter Cauliflower Rice (page 17) that has a little dried thyme and zested lemon stirred through.

CALORIES 447 | CARBOHYDRATES 1.3G | PROTEIN 36G | FAT 33G

4 SERVINGS **10m** PREP TIME **45m** COOK TIME

1 tablespoon lard

4 large chicken thighs (approx. 170g/6oz each)

1 large lemon, thinly sliced, pips removed

2 garlic cloves, very thinly sliced

4 sprigs fresh thyme, plus extra to serve

300ml (10fl oz) best-quality warm chicken stock

salt flakes, salt and freshly ground black pepper

If the chicken thighs you source aren't big enough for your liking, simply add more – there should be enough zingy glaze to brush over.

Preheat the oven to 200°C/180°C fan/400°F/gas mark 6.

Melt the lard in a deep-sided, ovenproof, non-stick pan over a medium–high heat. Season both sides of the chicken with a little salt. Fry the chicken thighs, skin side-down, for about 1–2 minutes until the skin turns golden and crispy. Turn and cook the undersides for another 3–4 minutes. Remove using tongs (or a slotted spoon) and set aside on a plate, leaving all the rendered fat and juices in the pan.

The pan will still be very hot, so remove it from the heat before adding the lemon slices, garlic and thyme. Stir well to quickly fry in the residual heat, then pour in the warm chicken stock. Return the chicken thighs to the pan, nestling in among the lemon slices, being careful not to wet the crispy skins.

Place in the oven for 35–40 minutes for the chicken to cook through sufficiently. A meat thermometer probe is useful here; the internal temperature should read 72°C (161.5°F) in the thickest part of the chicken. When done, remove from the oven. Use tongs or a slotted spoon to remove the chicken and lemon slices from the pan and set aside to keep warm while you finish the glaze.

Strain the stock and cooking juices into a small, clean pan. (Discard the garlic and thyme sprigs, they have done their job of infusing the stock.) Reduce over a high heat for approximately 8–10 minutes, until it boils down to a very thick and glossy glaze.

To serve, plate up the warm chicken and lemon, then use a pastry brush to simply brush the chicken skins with the deliciously zingy glaze. Season with salt flakes and freshly ground black pepper, and garnish with additional thyme.

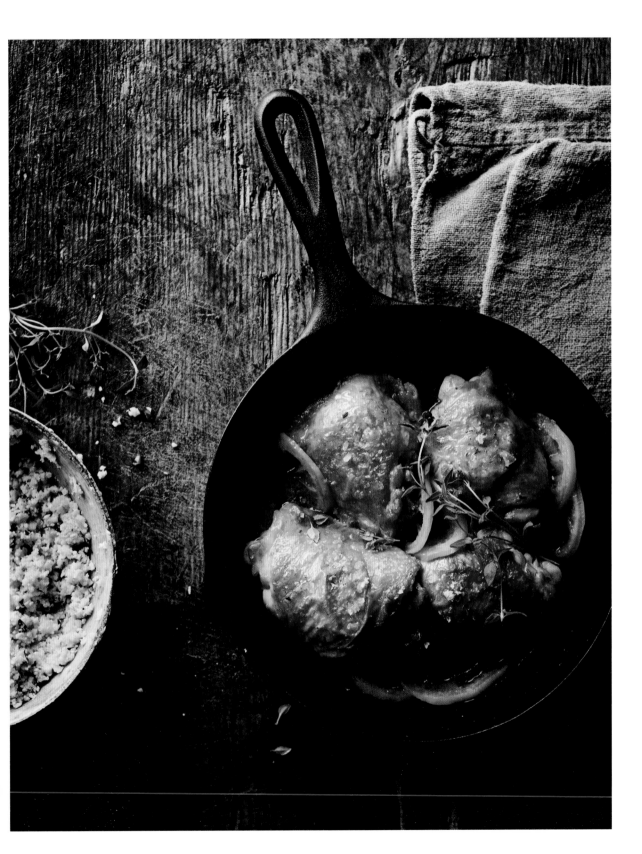

Chicken & Broccoli

with Paprika Bacon Butter

Minimal cleaning up, plenty of glorious broccoli and smoked fatty bacon lardons; this simple family chicken dinner boasts massive flavours thanks to the essential addition of smoked paprika. The red onion wedges offer wonderful little bites of sweetness in every mouthful and are truly delicious when roasted like this. *Pictured on page 70.*

 4 SERVINGS   **20m** PREP TIME   **40m** COOK TIME

CALORIES 657 | CARBOHYDRATES 8.7G | PROTEIN 49G | FAT 46G

8 chicken pieces (thighs and drumsticks), approx. 1.2kg (2lb 10oz) total weight

1 tablespoon smoked paprika

50g (1¾oz) unsalted butter

200g (7oz) smoked bacon lardons

450g (1lb) broccoli florets (approximately 2 medium heads)

1 red onion, cut into 8 wedges (see Tip)

salt flakes, salt and freshly ground black pepper

Keep the root end of the onion intact when cutting it into wedges, as this will ensure each wedge holds together when cooking.

Preheat the oven to 220°C/200°C fan/425°F/gas mark 7.

Season the chicken pieces on all sides with salt, freshly ground black pepper and half the smoked paprika. Get stuck in, using your hands to massage the seasoning into all the chicken pieces. Spread them out, skin side-up, on a large, greased roasting tray and place in the oven for 20 minutes.

In the meantime, melt the butter over a low heat in a non-stick pan and add the smoked bacon lardons. Add the remaining half tablespoon smoked paprika and gently cook until the lardons cook through.

Place the broccoli florets and red onion wedges into a large bowl and pour over the bacon-butter mixture, tossing well to evenly coat. (The butter may solidify a little, so do this just before the chicken's 20 minutes are up).

After the chicken has had its 20 minutes, remove it from the oven and reduce the temperature to 200°C/180°C fan/400°F/gas mark 6.

Use tongs to remove the partially cooked chicken pieces from the tray, setting them aside on a plate. Spread the broccoli mixture onto the tray, tossing it well in any rendered fat and juices from the chicken. Return the chicken pieces to the tray, nestling them in among the vegetables. If any juice ran from the chicken while it was set aside on the plate, drizzle this over the vegetables too. Return the tray to the oven for 20 minutes for the vegetables to roast and the chicken to sufficiently cook through. If in doubt, use a thermometer probe to check the thickest part of one thigh. It should read 72°C (161.5°F).

Season with salt flakes before tucking in.

Mediterranean Chicken
with Lemon & Oregano

6
SERVINGS

20m
PREP TIME

50m
COOK TIME

I love the Mediterranean flavours of this family dinner: cherry tomatoes, black olives, a dominant lemony element and fresh oregano. For maximum punch, please source the best-quality black olives that you can afford. Same for the tomatoes: ripe, organic and on the vine is the way to go. The fresh oregano I use to garnish at the end is an important flavour element, but the fresh kind may not always be available, so I encourage you to make the effort to source it before trying this dish (or simply grow your own!). *Pictured on page 70.*

CALORIES 480 | CARBOHYDRATES 4.3G | PROTEIN 33G | FAT 36G

6 large chicken thighs (approx. 170g/6oz each)

600g (1lb 5oz) cauliflower florets

1 teaspoon dried oregano

2 garlic cloves, very thinly sliced

2 lemons

100g (3½oz) cherry tomatoes, halved

50g (1¾oz) best-quality black olives, pitted and sliced

30g (1oz) unsalted butter

salt and freshly ground black pepper

To serve

salt flakes

small handful of fresh oregano leaves, roughly chopped

small handful of fresh flat-leaf parsley, roughly chopped

finely grated zest of 1 lemon

Preheat the oven to 220°C/200°C fan/425°F/gas mark 7.

Season all sides of the chicken thighs with salt and freshly ground black pepper and place them, skin side-up, in a large, deep roasting tray. Place in the oven for 20 minutes.

In the meantime, blitz the cauliflower florets in a food processor. Transfer to a large bowl and stir through the dried oregano, sliced garlic and the finely grated zest of 2 lemons. Slice the lemons in half and squeeze over the juice. Stir in the cherry tomatoes and olives.

Melt the butter in a small pan over a medium heat, then pour it over the cauliflower mixture. Season with salt and stir well. (The butter may solidify, so do this just before the chicken's 20 minutes are up.)

After the chicken has been in the oven for 20 minutes, remove it and reduce the temperature to 200°C/180°C fan/400°F/gas mark 6.

Use tongs or a slotted spoon to remove the partially cooked chicken thighs from the roasting tray and set aside. Tip the cauliflower mixture into the roasting tray and toss it in all in the juices.

Return the chicken thighs to the tray, nestling them into the cauliflower mixture. If any juice ran from the chicken while it was set aside on the plate, drizzle this over the cauliflower too. Return the dish to the oven for 20–25 minutes for the chicken to sufficiently cook through. If in doubt, use a thermometer probe to check the thickest part of one thigh. It should read 72°C (161.5°F). Give the cauli mix a stir halfway through to avoid the cauliflower on the edges burning.

To serve, season the dish with salt flakes, roughly chopped fresh oregano, chopped parsley and the finely grated zest of the third lemon.

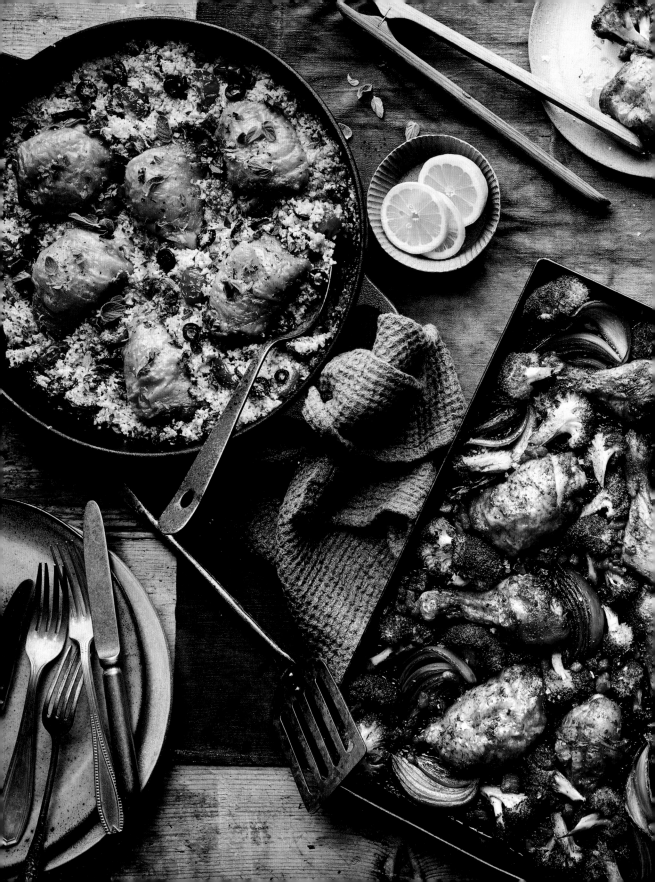

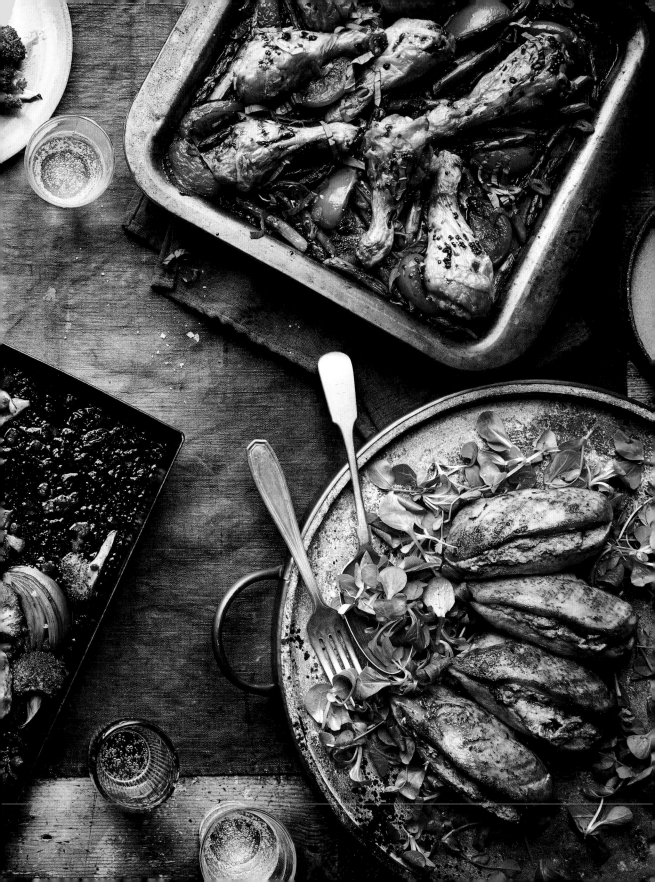

Chicken & Asparagus
with Balsamic Drizzle

This is fantastic midweek meal where chicken drumsticks are simply roasted with asparagus, tomatoes and garlic. You will especially love the dynamite balsamic reduction drizzled over at the end – it brings a sharpness that shapes the whole dish, and the fresh basil garnish finishes it off to perfection. All the flavours work so well together! Add more drumsticks if two per person doesn't seem realistic to you or you want more protein. *Pictured on page 71.*

4 SERVINGS | **10m** PREP TIME | **40m** COOK TIME

CALORIES 481 | CARBOHYDRATES 8.2G | PROTEIN 33G | FAT 34G

For the chicken and vegetables

8 large chicken drumsticks (approx. 165g/5¾oz each)

200g (7oz) fresh asparagus, cut into thirds

4 small–medium tomatoes, quartered

4 garlic cloves, very thinly sliced

2 teaspoons unsalted butter

salt flakes, salt and freshly ground black pepper

generous handful of fresh basil leaves, finely sliced, to serve

For the balsamic drizzle

100ml (3½fl oz) balsamic vinegar

2 teaspoons wholegrain mustard

Preheat the oven to 220°C/200°C fan/425°F/gas mark 7.

Season the drumsticks on all sides with salt and freshly ground black pepper. Spread out on a large, greased baking tray and place in the oven for 25 minutes.

Meanwhile, place the asparagus, tomatoes and garlic into a large bowl. Melt the butter in a small pan over a medium heat and pour over the vegetables. Season with salt and mix well to evenly coat. (The butter may solidify, so do this just before the chicken's 25 minutes are up).

After the chicken has been in the oven for 25 minutes, use tongs to remove the drumsticks from the tray (ensuring all the juices remain in the tray) and set the drumsticks aside on a plate. Spread the vegetables out on the tray, tossing them well in the juices. Return the drumsticks to the tray, nestling them in among the vegetables. If any juice ran from the chicken while it was set aside on the plate, drizzle this over the vegetables too. Return to the oven for 15 minutes.

In the meantime, place the balsamic vinegar and wholegrain mustard in a small pan over a moderately high heat. Whisk continuously until it reduces to a thick glaze. Keep your eye on it as this won't take long (and don't forget to turn on your extractor fan!).

Season the dish with salt flakes and drizzle over the balsamic reduction. Finish with sliced basil leaves and serve.

Pesto-stuffed Chicken Breasts

It's not easy doing something remarkable with chicken breasts: they can be somewhat underwhelming and easily dry out. To be honest, they are my least favourite cut and remind me of a life when I was still calorie-counting. However, their shape and size make them an ideal option to slice open and fill with a stuffing. The result is delicious and succulent! Serve with a salad or your choice of veg on the side. *Pictured on page 71.*

4 SERVINGS | **20m** PREP TIME | **40m** COOK TIME

CALORIES 353 | CARBOHYDRATES 2.2G | PROTEIN 41G | FAT 19G

4 large chicken breasts, skinless and deboned (approx. 210g/7½oz each)

1 teaspoon smoked paprika

2 teaspoons lard

100g (3½oz) full-fat cream cheese

40g (1½oz) Homemade Pesto (page 23)

30g (1oz) sun-dried tomatoes, drained and chopped very small

salt and freshly ground black pepper

Preheat the oven to 200°C/180°C fan/400°F/gas mark 6.

Remove the chicken breasts from their packaging and pat dry with kitchen paper. Scatter over the smoked paprika on all sides of the chicken, using your hands to rub it in evenly.

Melt the lard in a large non-stick pan over a very high heat and brown the chicken breasts on all sides. You want to get some good colour on them, without burning them. Remove from the heat and set aside.

Once they are cool enough to handle, make a deep incision in the side of each breast. This is best done by placing your hand firmly down on the breast and using a very sharp knife to cut a pocket three-quarters of the way through the side. Remember, you are still working with partially raw chicken, so be mindful when handling it.

Make the stuffing by simply combining the cream cheese, pesto and sun-dried tomatoes in a small bowl. Season with salt and freshly ground black pepper. Spoon the pesto mixture into the chicken pockets and place the stuffed chicken breasts on a greased baking tray.

Cook in the oven for 25–30 minutes or until the chicken has cooked through sufficiently. Serve with a salad or your choice of vegetables.

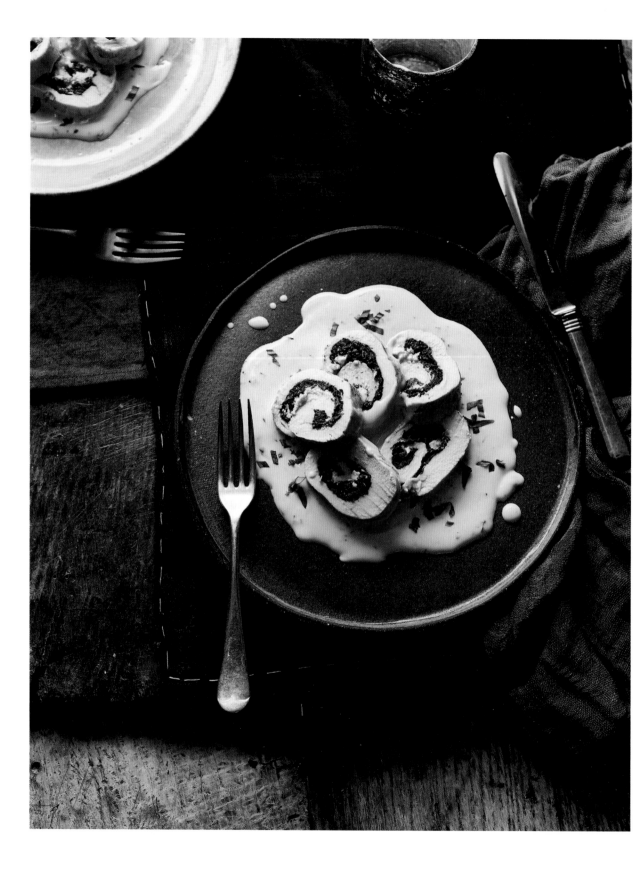

'Date Night' Chicken

with Tarragon Yogurt Sauce

2 SERVINGS

30m PREP TIME

45m COOK TIME

I called this dish 'date night' chicken as it requires some reasonable effort that I am just not sure the kids will appreciate! The sauce is so tasty and you could serve it over regular grilled chicken thighs if you are not up for all the prep involved in making the pinwheel parcels. I would serve such a rich dish with a very simple side, like steamed greens or a fresh salad, but that glorious sauce deserves to be mopped up, so maybe Creamy Cauliflower Mash (page 16) would work too.

CALORIES 651 | CARBOHYDRATES 3.5G | PROTEIN 65G | FAT 41G

2 teaspoons unsalted butter

120g (4¼oz) baby spinach leaves, little stalks removed

2 large chicken breasts, skinless and deboned (approx. 210g/ 7½oz each – source the largest breasts you can find, as they will be much easier to work with)

pinch of ground coriander

50g (1¾oz) full-fat feta cheese

2 teaspoons lard

salt flakes (optional), salt and freshly ground black pepper

For the tarragon yogurt sauce

65ml (2¼fl oz) dry white wine

generous handful of fresh tarragon leaves, chopped

65g (2¼oz) full-fat plain yogurt

65ml (2¼fl oz) double cream

½ tablespoon Dijon mustard

Preheat the oven to 200°C/180°C fan/400°F/gas mark 6.

Melt the butter in a large non-stick pan over a medium–high heat. Add the baby spinach, cooking until completely wilted and all the moisture has evaporated. While stirring, mash the spinach. Remove and set aside.

Place your hand firmly down on each chicken breast and use a very sharp knife to cut a pocket three-quarters of the way through the side. Open each breast up and place between 2 sheets of parchment paper. Sliced side-up, pound the thicker pieces using the flat side of a meat mallet until each breast is thin and even. Don't pound them to shreds!

Peel off the top sheet of parchment. Season the flattened breasts with salt and coriander. Spread the spinach onto each breast and finely crumble the feta cheese over the spinach. Tuck in the sides of the chicken, then roll each one up tightly, ensuring none of the filling bulges out. Wrap each roll in a sheet of kitchen foil. Place both parcels on a baking tray and cook in the oven for 35 minutes. When cool enough to handle, discard the foil. You will be left with 2 cooked chicken logs.

Melt the lard in a non-stick pan over a medium–high heat and brown the chicken logs on all sides, handling them very gently. This step is optional, but it adds a lovely caramelized flavour. Set aside to keep warm.

To make the sauce, add the wine and three-quarters of the chopped tarragon to a small pan over a medium heat and reduce by two-thirds. Reduce the heat to low and whisk in the yogurt, cream and mustard. The sauce should be thick enough, so keep it on the heat to stay warm.

Use a sharp knife to slice the chicken logs into pinwheels and serve with the sauce. Season with salt flakes (if needed) and freshly ground black pepper. Scatter over the remaining chopped tarragon leaves.

Fresh Green Chicken Curry

4 SERVINGS · **20m** PREP TIME · **40m** COOK TIME

I use succulent skinless and deboned chicken thighs for this lovely curry. Thighs are far superior to breasts for this type of cooking as they won't dry out after all the simmering. The flavour of my quick homemade green paste is fresh and fragrant, and you will taste the love and effort you have put in. I love this over Garlic Butter Cauliflower Rice (page 17), as pictured. If you choose to serve it this way, stir a little chopped fresh coriander through the cooked cauliflower rice to enhance the flavour.

CALORIES 545 | CARBOHYDRATES 7.1G | PROTEIN 42G | FAT 38G

For the green chilli paste

3–4 green chillies, deseeded and chopped

½ onion, roughly chopped

thumb-sized piece of ginger, peeled and chopped

2 garlic cloves, roughly chopped

1 lemongrass stalk, roughly chopped (discard the hard outer layer)

1 teaspoon fish sauce

1 teaspoon ground coriander

½ teaspoon ground cumin

handful of fresh coriander leaves

very generous crack of black pepper

finely grated zest and juice of 1 lime

For the curry

8 chicken thighs (skinless, deboned), chopped (approx. 850g/1lb 14oz) in total

1 tablespoon coconut oil

generous squeeze of lime juice, plus extra to serve

4 spring onions, thickly sliced

400ml (14fl oz) full-fat coconut milk

2 kaffir lime leaves (fresh or dried)

fish sauce (optional)

salt

1 red chilli, sliced, and a small handful of chopped fresh coriander, to serve

For the paste, simply blitz all the ingredients in a mini food processor/food chopper with 2 tablespoons cold water. Stop intermittently to scrape down the sides of the bowl. Blitz until you have a smooth puree. Set aside.

To make the curry, season the chicken pieces with a little salt. Melt the coconut oil in a large non-stick pan or wok over a high heat. Add the chicken and fry until golden and caramelized on the outside before removing and setting aside on a plate (see Tip).

Once all the chicken has been removed, reduce the heat to medium. Deglaze the pan with a generous squeeze of lime juice, scraping the bottom to loosen any chicken bits that are stuck. Tip in the chilli paste, along with the spring onions, and cook for 5–6 minutes, stirring regularly.

Add the coconut milk and kaffir lime leaves and cook until the mixture has thickened and reduced by half. Scrape down the sides of the pan or wok with a silicone spatula as the mixture reduces.

Return the chicken pieces to the pan – along with any resting juices – and cook over a medium heat until you have a thick, creamy curry and you are satisfied that the chicken has safely cooked through (cut open one piece to check: it should not be pink).

Taste and adjust the seasoning with salt or a very small dash of fish sauce. If you feel it could do with a little more acidity, squeeze over a little extra lime juice if you have another lime kicking about.

Serve the curry topped with red chilli and coriander.

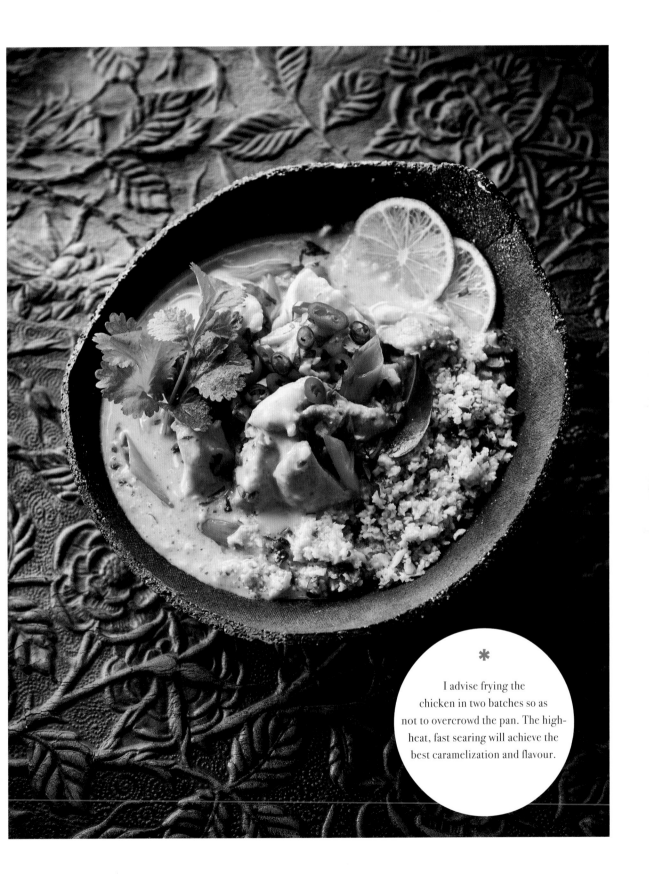

*

I advise frying the
chicken in two batches so as
not to overcrowd the pan. The high-
heat, fast searing will achieve the
best caramelization and flavour.

Fresh & Light Asian Steak Salad

This fast and simple steak salad offers strong, fresh Asian flavours with every forkful and comes in at just 6.8g carbs per generous serving. You can use any steak that fits your budget, but I would recommend a leaner cut since the steak is enjoyed in a salad and too much fat present in a chilled steak may congeal unpleasantly. While this lean dish may go against the high-fat lifestyle of keto, I sometimes desire something a little less 'heavy', especially in summer. Fear not, though; it will not disappoint when it comes to flavour!

CALORIES 308 | CARBOHYDRATES 6.8G | PROTEIN 39G | FAT 13G

 2 SERVINGS **20m** PREP TIME **10m** COOK TIME

2 large cucumbers

½ small red onion, thinly sliced

2 spring onions, sliced

½ lemongrass stalk, finely chopped (discard the hard outer layer)

small handful of fresh mint leaves, finely chopped

small handful of fresh coriander leaves, finely chopped

juice of 1 lime, plus extra to serve

2 teaspoons rice wine vinegar

1 tablespoon fish sauce

2 rump steaks (approximately 160g/5¾oz each)

2 teaspoons lard (or coconut oil)

salt

1 red chilli, sliced, plus extra to serve

Trim the ends of the cucumbers and halve each one lengthways. Use a vegetable peeler along the length of each piece to create thin ribbons. Dice the centre bits very small.

Combine the red onion, cucumber ribbons and diced centres, spring onions, lemongrass, mint and coriander in a large, wide-bottomed serving bowl. Pour over the lime juice, rice wine vinegar and fish sauce and combine well to evenly marinate (see Tip). Set aside while you cook the steaks, but give it a good toss every now and then to ensure even marinating.

To cook the steaks, start by patting them dry using kitchen paper.

Season on all sides with a little salt. Melt the lard (or coconut oil) in a non-stick pan over a high heat. Fry the steaks until done to your liking, then remove from the pan and set aside to rest for at least 5 minutes.

Place a colander over a bowl and tip the cucumber mixture into the colander, draining well, but reserving all the flavoured juice. Plate up the cucumber mix in a larger sharing bowl (or divide between 2 plates).

Slice the rested steak into thin strips and serve on top of the cucumber salad. Drizzle the reserved marinating juices over the top and scatter over the sliced red chilli.

Have extra limes and chillies handy (if needed) and enjoy immediately.

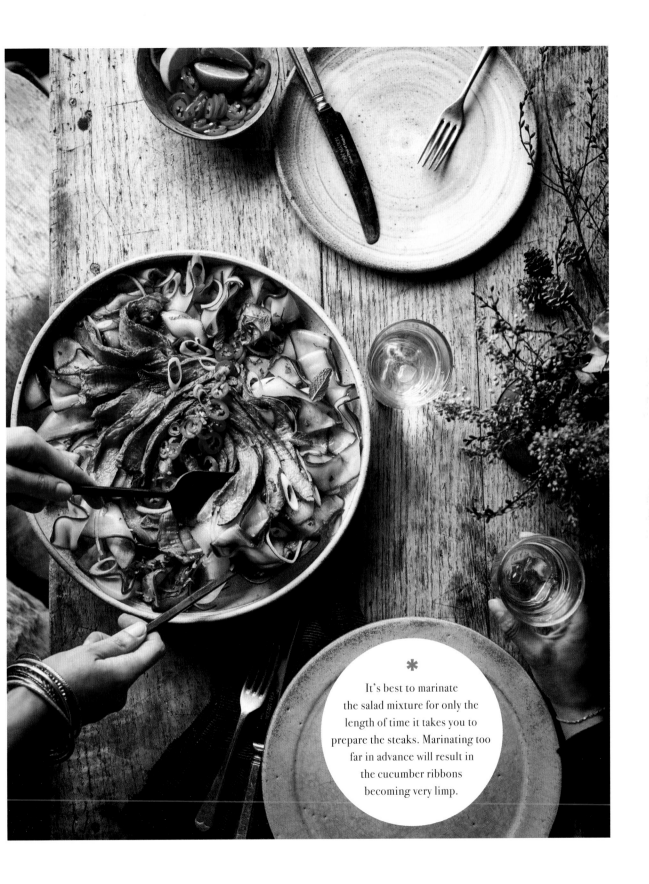

*

It's best to marinate
the salad mixture for only the
length of time it takes you to
prepare the steaks. Marinating too
far in advance will result in
the cucumber ribbons
becoming very limp.

Quick & Easy Phở Bò

This is my quick and easy version of Vietnamese phở (pronounced 'fuh', not 'foh' or 'foo') using courgette noodles to sneak some lovely vegetables in. Don't be too intimidated by the long list of ingredients here, you likely have most of them in your pantry already. The size of your steak will be your own personal choice. The macros are calculated on using two medium-sized rump steaks (180g/6½oz each) – but there is no judgement here if you decide to Go Bigger!

2 SERVINGS | **20m** PREP TIME | **15m** COOK TIME

CALORIES 427 | CARBOHYDRATES 6.1G | PROTEIN 47G | FAT 22G

2 whole star anise

2 whole cloves

2 cinnamon sticks

2 teaspoons whole black peppercorns

2 teaspoons whole coriander seeds

750ml (25fl oz) best-quality beef stock

1 thumb-size piece of ginger, peeled and sliced

1 garlic clove, sliced

1 teaspoon lard

2 medium rump steaks (approx. 180g/6½oz each)

2 teaspoons fish sauce

juice of 1 lime

200g (7oz) courgette noodles (see Tip)

To serve

40g (1½oz) beansprouts, rinsed well, then drained

2 spring onions, sliced

small handful of fresh mint leaves

small handful of fresh coriander leaves

1 red chilli, thinly sliced

Heat a dry, deep, non-stick pan over a medium heat and toast the star anise, cloves, cinnamon sticks, peppercorns and coriander seeds until fragrant. Pour in the beef stock and add the ginger and garlic. Bring the mixture to a simmer for 2–3 minutes, then remove the pan from the heat and set aside for 10 minutes to allow the aromatics to infuse the stock.

In the meantime, melt the lard in a separate pan over a very high heat and sear the steaks until browned on all sides and done to your liking. I prefer them rare on the inside for this dish as the hot broth will later (ever so slightly) cook them further. Remove from the pan and set aside to rest.

Strain the fragrant broth through a fine mesh sieve (discarding all the whole spices, ginger and garlic) into a clean pan and reheat gently. Stir in the fish sauce and squeeze in the lime juice.

Divide the courgette noodles between 2 warm bowls and pour in the hot, fragrant broth.

Slice the steaks thinly and add to the bowls on top of the noodles. Top each bowl with beansprouts, spring onions, fresh herbs and chilli slices, then serve.

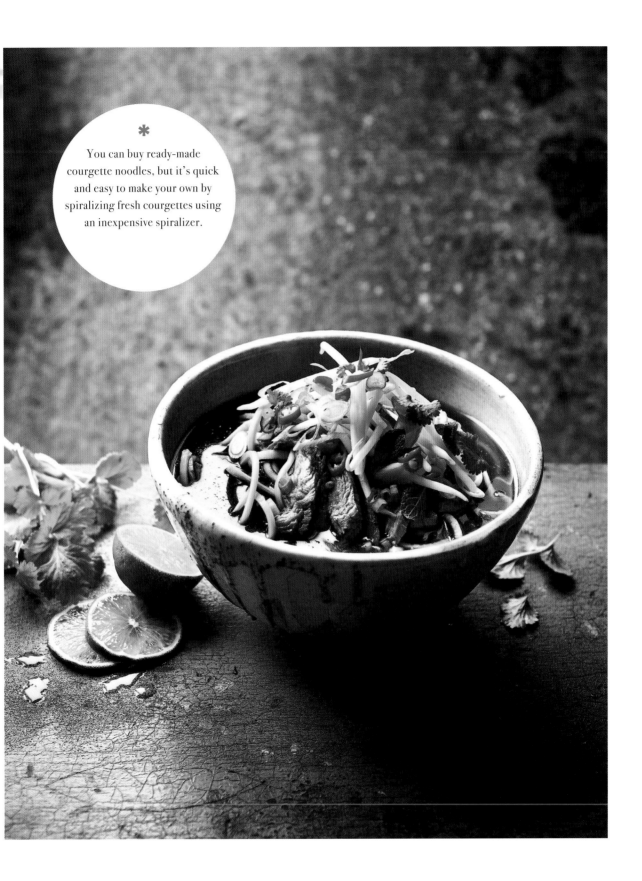

You can buy ready-made
courgette noodles, but it's quick
and easy to make your own by
spiralizing fresh courgettes using
an inexpensive spiralizer.

Chilli con Carne

This is such a comforting bowl of spicy goodness and I love whipping it up during the chilly months. I packed in some vegetables to replace the traditional red kidney beans while keeping the carbs as low as possible. It's finished with all the authentic toppings – soured cream, grated cheese, parsley and fresh red chillies. I tuck into my bowl with a spoon and don't even miss the tortilla or rice, but if you feel you want to enjoy it with a base, it will go beautifully over the Garlic Butter Cauliflower Rice (page 17). *Pictured on page 84.*

4 SERVINGS | **15m** PREP TIME | **1hr** COOK TIME

CALORIES 623 | CARBOHYDRATES 8.8G | PROTEIN 38G | FAT 47G

---

2 teaspoons lard

½ medium onion, diced small

1 green pepper, diced small

100g (3½oz) mushrooms, chopped small

3 garlic cloves, thinly sliced

2 tablespoons ground cumin

2 teaspoons ground coriander

1 teaspoon cayenne pepper (adjust to your liking)

1 tablespoon red wine vinegar

650g (1lb 7oz) minced beef, 20 per cent fat

400g (14oz) chopped tomatoes, canned or fresh

300ml (10fl oz) best-quality beef stock

salt and freshly ground black pepper

To serve

100g (3½oz) soured cream

60g (2¼oz) extra-mature full-fat Cheddar cheese, grated

handful of fresh flat-leaf parsley, finely chopped

1–2 red chillies, finely sliced

Melt the lard in a large non-stick pan over a medium heat. Add the diced onion and green pepper and cook until they have softened a little. Add the mushrooms and garlic and cook until the mushrooms release all their moisture and the vegetables begin to brown and caramelize (stir regularly to avoid the garlic burning). Add the cumin, coriander and cayenne pepper and stir well to combine.

Deglaze the pan with the red wine vinegar. Once all the liquid cooks out, tip in all the minced beef and increase the heat, stirring continuously, until the mince evenly browns.

Tip in the chopped tomatoes and beef stock and bring to the boil. Immediately reduce to a low–medium heat and partially cover with a lid, cooking for about 30 minutes. Check on it regularly to stir.

After 30 minutes, remove the lid completely and cook for an additional 15–20 minutes, stirring occasionally to ensure the mixture is not sticking to the bottom of the pan. It will be ready once the mixture is thick and chunky and free from any wateriness or excess liquid. Taste and season accordingly with salt and freshly ground black pepper.

Divide between 4 bowls and top each with soured cream, grated Cheddar, chopped parsley and sliced red chillies.

Monnie's Meatball Marinara

Meatballs are always a crowd-pleaser! Here, I enhance high-fat minced beef with a generous dollop of my Homemade Pesto (page 23), adding another flavour dimension, and add ground chia for binding. The meatballs are browned in batches, then slowly cooked in my Roasted Tomato Marinara Sauce (page 23). I love these over Buttered Courgetti (page 17). The prep time excludes the making of the Pesto and Marinara, so please keep that in mind when planning. *Pictured on page 85.*

4 SERVINGS   **20m** PREP TIME   **40m** COOK TIME

CALORIES 762 | CARBOHYDRATES 7.9G | PROTEIN 42G | FAT 60G

650g (1lb 7oz) minced beef, 20 per cent fat

65g (2½oz) Homemade Pesto (page 23)

30g (1oz) ground chia seeds

1 large egg, whisked well

2 teaspoons lard

60ml (4 tablespoons) dry red wine

450g (1lb) Roasted Tomato Marinara Sauce (page 23)

½ teaspoon dried oregano

To serve

chilli-infused olive oil (optional)

60g (2¼oz) extra-mature full-fat Cheddar, grated

30g (1oz) Parmesan cheese, finely grated

small handful of fresh flat-leaf parsley, finely chopped

salt and freshly ground black pepper

Combine the minced beef, pesto, ground chia and whisked egg in a large bowl. Season with salt and pepper and mix well until thoroughly combined.

Form the mixture into small, compact ping-pong-sized balls using your hands and a spoon. Set them aside on a tray.

Melt the lard in a large, deep, non-stick pan over a high heat. Brown the meatballs in three batches until golden and browned on the outside. Turn them gently to avoid them falling apart. After each batch is done, set them aside on a plate before browning the next batch. You don't need them to cook through at this stage; this step is just to get that lovely brown crust on the outside, which adds flavour.

Once all the meatballs have been browned, pour out the rendered fat, but do not discard it. Add the red wine to the pan, scraping the bottom to loosen any stuck bits. Cook until the wine has completely cooked out and evaporated.

Reduce the heat to medium and add the Marinara Sauce and dried oregano, then lightly whisk in the fat you set aside earlier. Return the meatballs to the pan, nestling them in the sauce. Cook for 20 minutes over this medium heat, carefully turning the meatballs in the sauce every now and then. This will ensure they are cooked all the way through as the sauce reduces and thickens.

Serve over Buttered Courgetti or your favourite base. Season as needed with salt and freshly ground black pepper. If you like a kick, drizzle over a little chilli-infused oil and top with the grated cheese and chopped parsley.

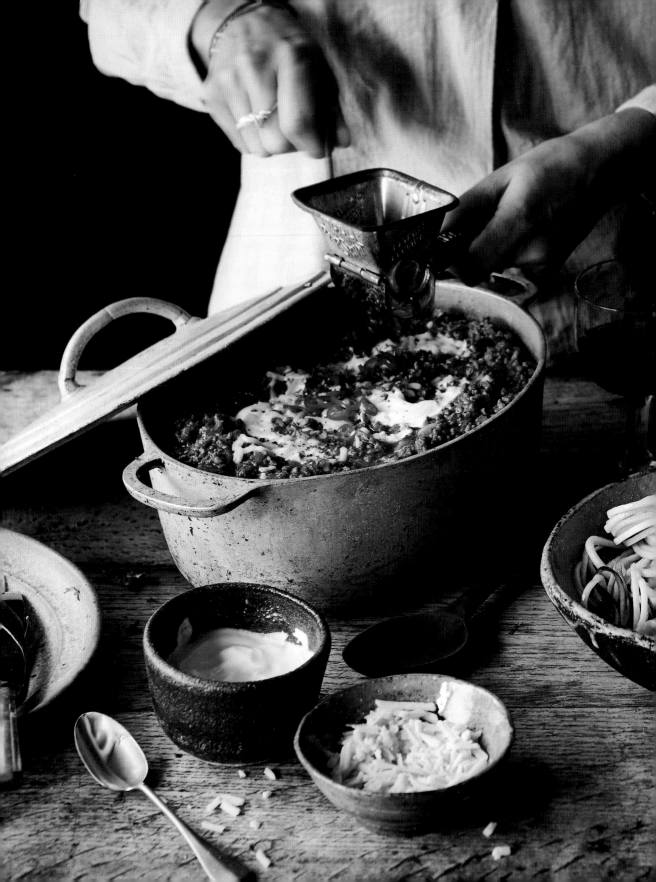

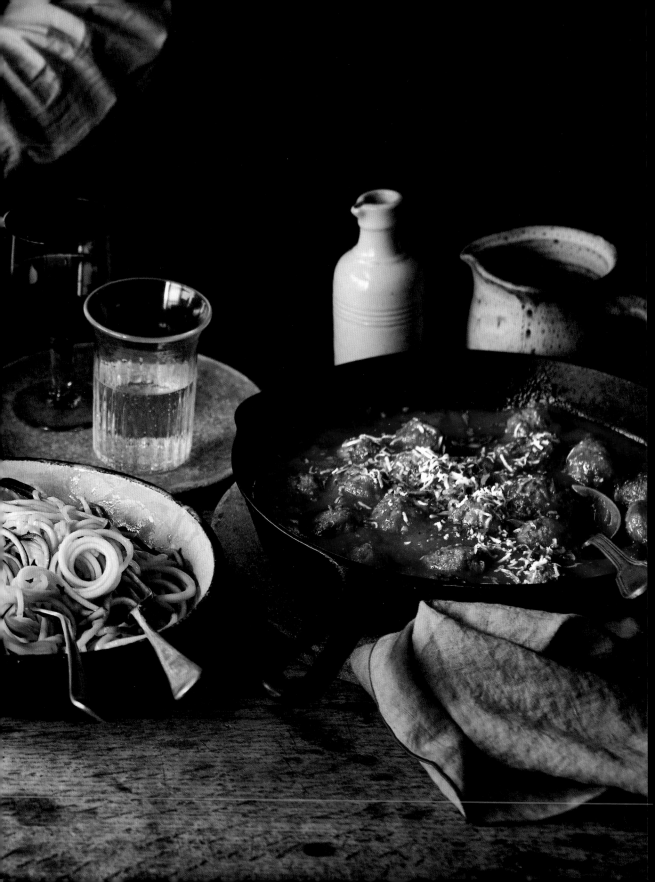

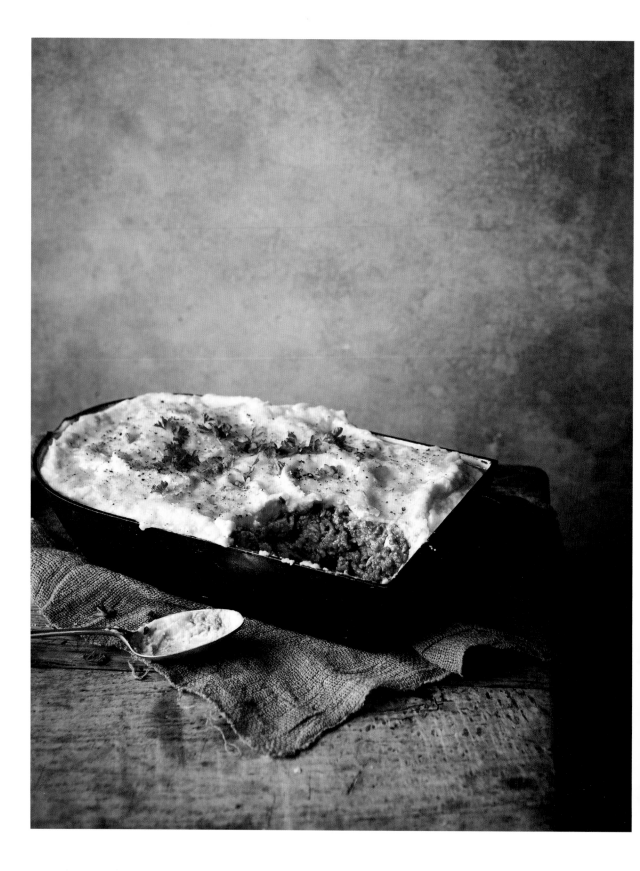

Spicy Cottage Pie

When I was young, a humble cottage pie was one of the first things I remember learning to make. I guess because it's dead easy and the hearty, familiar flavours make it such a popular dinner option. Here, I replace the traditional potato topping with creamy mashed cauliflower (boasting a hint of mustard) and add cayenne pepper to the beef to give it some kick. Adjust the amount of cayenne pepper to your liking, or leave it out altogether if you are cooking for the kids. Enjoy this with a lovely fresh salad on the side.

4 SERVINGS | **20m** PREP TIME | **40m** COOK TIME

CALORIES 543 | CARBOHYDRATES 9.7G | PROTEIN 34G | FAT 40G

For the cauliflower mustard mash

500g (1lb 2oz) cauliflower florets

50g (1¾oz) full-fat cream cheese

1 tablespoon Dijon mustard

2 teaspoons unsalted butter

salt and ground white pepper

For the cottage pie

2 teaspoons lard

1 onion, finely chopped

120g (4½oz) mushrooms, finely chopped

2 garlic cloves, very thinly sliced

2 tablespoons red wine vinegar

500g (1lb 2oz) minced beef, 20 per cent fat

½ teaspoon dried thyme

2 teaspoons cayenne pepper (or chilli powder)

200g (7oz) chopped tomatoes, canned or fresh

50g (1¾oz) extra-mature full-fat Cheddar cheese, grated

salt flakes, salt and freshly ground black pepper

small handful of fresh flat-leaf parsley, finely chopped, to serve

Preheat the oven to 220°C/200°C fan/425°F/gas mark 7.

Make the cauliflower mustard mash topping by following the method on page 16 and adding the mustard at the same time as the cream cheese. Set aside, keeping warm.

Meanwhile, melt the lard in a large, non-stick pan over a medium heat. Cook the onion until softened and partially caramelized. Add the mushrooms and garlic and cook until the mushrooms have softened and caramelized. Keep stirring to avoid the garlic burning.

Deglaze the pan with the red wine vinegar. Cook until the vinegar cooks out, then tip in all the minced beef. Add the dried thyme and cayenne pepper (or chilli powder). Continue to cook until the minced beef browns evenly. Add the chopped tomatoes and reduce the heat to moderately low. Cook until all the liquid cooks out and you are left with a thick, chunky mixture. Taste to check seasoning and add salt if needed. Transfer to a suitably sized dish and spread over the warm cauliflower topping.

Scatter the grated Cheddar cheese over the top and place the dish on a tray (to avoid any bubbling over). Bake until the cheese bubbles and browns, approximately 15 minutes.

Once done, season with salt flakes and freshly ground black pepper. Scatter over the chopped parsley and serve.

Rib-eye Steaks

with Chimichurri

6 SERVINGS

15m PREP TIME

10m COOK TIME

Every year, I do a bit of private cheffing over the Queens and Wimbledon Championships for my favourite athlete. It has become a tradition that my husband joins me for a day, and we treat the team to a *braai* (barbecue). I always ensure there is steak and chimichurri on the spread. Here, the chimichurri is drizzled over sliced rib-eye (a glorious, fatty cut), but you could easily have this with a whole, sliced fillet or any other steak. A little chimichurri goes a long way: use it sparingly to avoid overshadowing the beautiful flavour of the meat.

CALORIES 548 | CARBOHYDRATES 1.4G | PROTEIN 50G | FAT 37G

For the rib-eye steaks

6 rib-eye steaks (approximately 200g/7oz each), ideally left uncovered in the refrigerator overnight – see method)

½ teaspoon dried oregano

salt and freshly ground black pepper

For the chimichurri

15g (½oz) fresh flat-leaf parsley, leaves only

1½ tablespoons fresh oregano, leaves only

2 garlic cloves, roughly chopped

1 tablespoon red wine vinegar

pinch of dried chilli flakes

50ml (1¾fl oz) olive oil

Six large rib-eyes could easily feed 8–10 people as part of a barbecue spread, but for the sake of the macros here, I've stuck to six (hungry) people!

This dish takes 25 minutes to throw together, but you really should start the day before. Remove the steaks from their packaging and place on a cooling rack set over a tray. Keep uncovered in the refrigerator overnight. Remove the steaks from the refrigerator 30 minutes before cooking.

Season both sides of the steaks with salt and freshly ground black pepper. Scatter over the dried oregano and use your hands to rub the steaks with the seasoning.

Once your coals are ready, grill the steaks, flipping them every 15–20 seconds (just like Heston taught us) until a dark crust forms on the outside and they are done to your liking. Remove the steaks from the pan and set aside to rest for at least 10 minutes. If you are doing this indoors, melt a little lard in a griddle pan and fry over a high heat in the same manner.

To make the chimichurri, simply add the parsley and oregano leaves to a mini food processor/food chopper. Add the garlic and red wine vinegar and blitz well. Be sure to scrape down the sides of the jug. Stir in the chilli flakes and olive oil and season with salt and freshly ground black pepper.

Slice the rested rib-eye into thin strips and serve with the chimichurri.

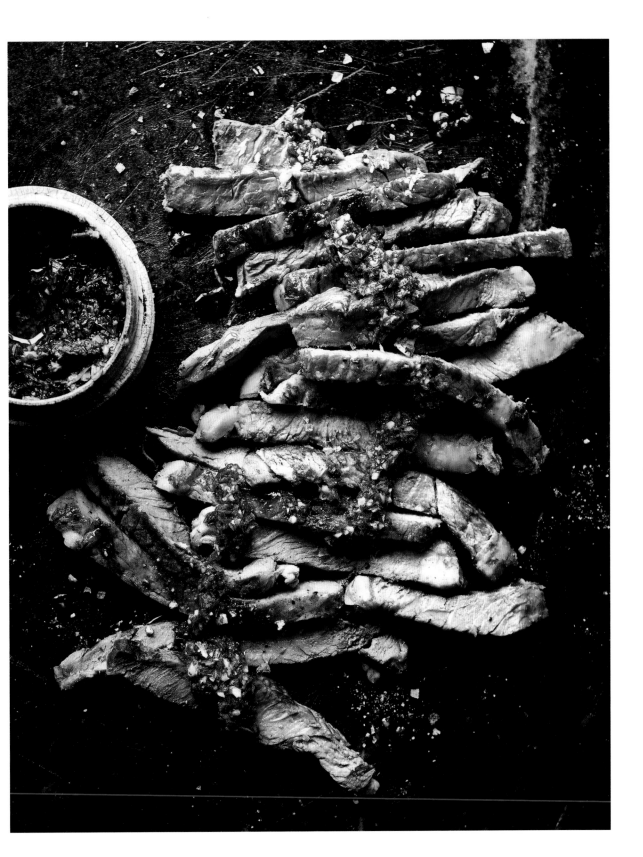

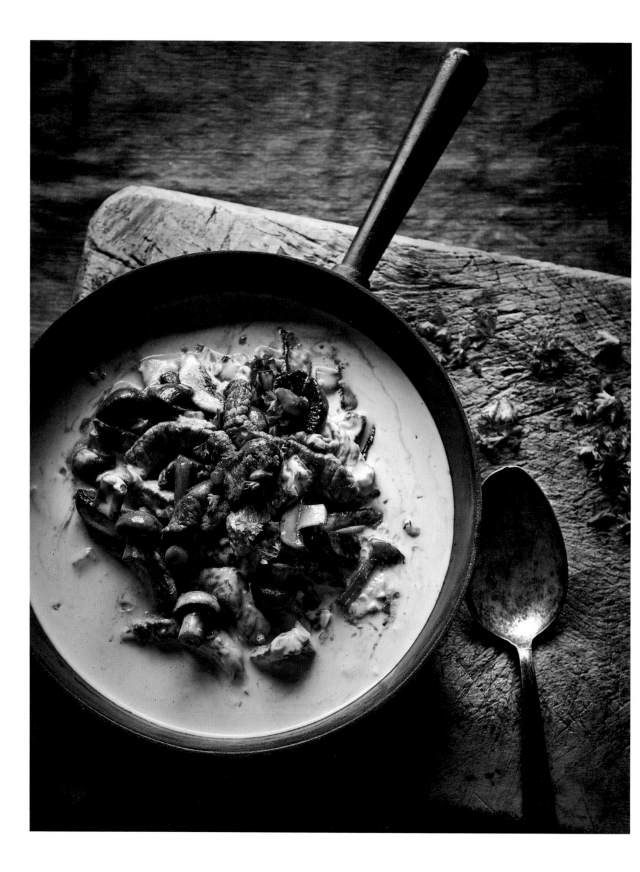

Ultimate Beef Stroganoff

This is my version of beef stroganoff, which doesn't result in overcooked beef strips. It's rich, sharp, creamy and simply delicious over Buttered Courgetti or Garlic Butter Cauliflower Rice (page 17). It yields two generous servings, so it's likely one of you could be looking forward to leftovers the next day …

 2 SERVINGS   **15m** PREP TIME   **35m** COOK TIME

CALORIES 694 | CARBOHYDRATES 7.8G | PROTEIN 36G | FAT 57G

2 rump steaks (approximately 140g/5oz each)

30g (1oz) unsalted butter

½ onion, finely chopped

2 cloves garlic, crushed

140g (5oz) mushrooms, thickly sliced

60ml (4 tablespoons) dry white wine

150ml (5fl oz) best-quality beef stock

150ml (5fl oz) double cream

1 teaspoon Dijon mustard

salt flakes, salt and freshly ground black pepper

small handful of fresh flat-leaf parsley, finely chopped, to serve

Work in batches. An overcrowded pan will lose heat and the steaks will simmer in their own juices. You need high-heat, fast searing to brown the outside and achieve the best flavour.

Season the steaks on all sides with salt, then slice into thin strips.

Melt half the butter in a large, deep, non-stick pan or wok over a very high heat. Sear the steak strips in the hot pan until browned and caramelized (see Tip).

Use tongs or a slotted spoon to remove the beef strips from the pan and set aside on a plate, ensuring all the butter, fat and juices remain in the pan. Reduce the heat and add the onion and garlic, cooking them gently until softened. Add the mushrooms and the remaining butter and cook until the mushrooms brown and caramelize.

Deglaze the pan with the wine, scraping the bottom of the pan to loosen any bits that have stuck. Once the wine evaporates and cooks out, pour in the stock. Cook until the stock reduces by more than two-thirds. Add the cream and mustard and continue to cook over a medium heat until the sauce thickens and reduces further, whisking if necessary.

Return the steak strips to the pan along with any resting juices that ran while they were set aside. Gently warm through for a minute or two.

Season with salt flakes and freshly ground black pepper, then scatter over the chopped parsley and serve.

Bacon & Mushroom Garlic Pizza

The dough for this pizza is made from a combination of almond flour and cheese. It may be a little tricky to get right, but once you master it, it will be your go-to when the craving for pizza hits! For those of you keeping track of your calories, you may want to clap eyes on the nutritional breakdown for this whopper. The pizza (with these toppings) is very rich, so I would advise sharing one between two people and enjoying it with a lovely fresh salad on the side.

 2 SERVINGS

 20m PREP TIME

 20m COOK TIME

PER ½ PIZZA | CALORIES 980 | CARBOHYDRATES 10G | PROTEIN 54G | FAT 78G

100g (3½oz) almond flour

¼ teaspoon salt

1 teaspoon garlic powder

60g (2¼oz) full-fat cream cheese

260g (9¼oz) grated pizza mozzarella (see Tip)

1 large egg, whisked well

150g (5½oz) smoked bacon lardons

50g (1¾oz) mushrooms, sliced

1 garlic clove, very thinly sliced

90g (3¼oz) Roasted Tomato Marinara Sauce (see page 23)

salt flakes and freshly ground black pepper

small handful of fresh flat-leaf parsley, finely chopped, to serve

If you choose to use fresh mozzarella, chop the balls into smaller pieces and drain off excess liquid after melting, otherwise your dough will be far too wet to work with.

Preheat the oven to 220°C/200°C fan/425°F/gas mark 7.

Combine the almond flour, salt and garlic powder in a bowl.

Place the cream cheese and 170g (6oz) of the grated mozzarella in a wide-bottomed, microwave-friendly bowl. Heat in the microwave on high for 90 seconds until the cheese has completely melted (see Tip).

Immediately tip the melted cheese into the bowl of almond flour mix and use a wooden spoon to vigorously combine. Add the whisked egg and continue to mix until the mixture comes together as a sticky dough. Allow to cool for 5 minutes, then place the ball of dough between 2 sheets of parchment paper. Use a rolling pin to roll it out into a large, circular shape to make your pizza base. Peel off the top layer of parchment and slide the base onto a large baking tray or pizza stone.

Bake in the preheated oven for 10 minutes, rotating halfway through.

In the meantime, prepare the toppings. Cook the bacon lardons in a non-stick pan over a medium heat. Once they start releasing all their fat and juices, add the mushrooms and sliced garlic. Continue to cook, stirring regularly, until the bacon crisps a little and the mushrooms have caramelized. In a separate pan, heat the Roasted Tomato Marinara Sauce until it thickens and any excess wateriness cooks out.

Remove the pizza from the oven and spoon the tomato sauce evenly over the base. Scatter over most of the remaining 90g (3¼oz) grated mozzarella, then scatter over the cooked bacon and mushroom mixture. Cover with the remainder of the mozzarella and return the pizza to the oven for an additional 5–6 minutes. Remove and season with salt and pepper. Scatter over the chopped parsley and serve.

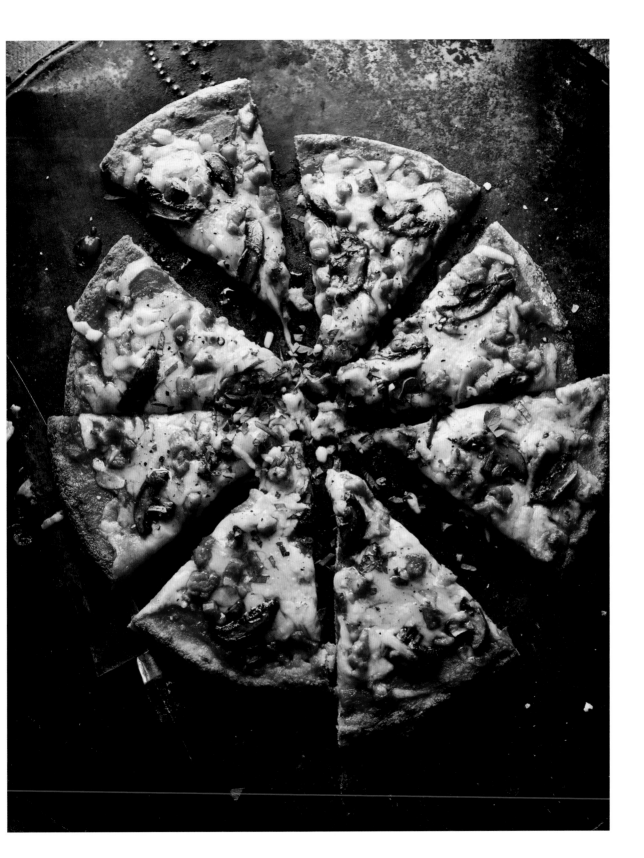

Pork Belly

with Red Onion Relish & Keto Gravy

A fantastic pork belly, with a simply delicious gravy, that will happily feed five people. The pickled red onion and herb relish is a beautiful, acidic accompaniment that really steals the show! The whole lot comes in at only 7.7g carbs per serving and makes for a show-stopping Sunday lunch. Serve alongside Celeriac Dauphinoise (page 114), Creamy Cauliflower Mash (page 16) or any other side vegetable that will benefit from all that tasty, thick gravy.

5 SERVINGS | **15m** PREP TIME | **3½hrs** COOK TIME

CALORIES 630 | CARBOHYDRATES 7.7G | PROTEIN 46G | FAT 45G

For the pickled red onion

1 red onion, very thinly sliced

3 tablespoons red wine vinegar

handful of fresh mint leaves, finely chopped

handful of fresh flat-leaf parsley, finely chopped

For the pork belly and gravy

1.1kg (2lb 7oz) boneless pork belly, skin scored (ideally removed from packaging and left, uncovered, in the refrigerator overnight)

generous pinch of salt flakes

2 teaspoons fennel seeds, lightly crushed with a pestle and mortar

2 onions, very thinly sliced

3 cloves garlic, very thinly sliced

1 tablespoon white wine vinegar

700ml (1¼ pints) warm best-quality chicken stock

The emulsification of the rendered pork fat and chicken stock will make your gravy thick and glossy. It needs to be made just before serving as the fat may split if left standing too long.

Place the sliced red onions in a bowl and pour over the red wine vinegar. Toss well to coat. Leave to pickle, stirring occasionally.

Preheat the oven to 240°C/220°C fan/475°F/gas mark 9.

Pat the pork belly dry using kitchen paper. Scatter the salt flakes over the skin, pressing them into the scored incisions. Place the belly in a deep casserole dish lined with parchment paper. Place in the oven for 25–30 minutes to get the skin puffed up.

Remove the casserole from the oven. Remove the pork and discard the parchment paper. Reduce the oven temperature to 160°C/140°C fan/325°F/gas mark 3. Scatter the fennel seeds over the puffed-up skin, using a teaspoon to work them into the scored incisions.

Place the onions, garlic, white wine vinegar and warm chicken stock into the casserole dish, then gently place the pork on top, ensuring the stock does not splash onto the crispy skin. Cook, uncovered, for 1 hour. After 1 hour, add 200ml (7fl oz) hot water to the casserole and return to the oven for an additional 2 hours.

After the full 3 hours, carefully lift the pork belly from the casserole and wrap the bottom in foil, keeping the skin exposed. Set aside to rest. Tip the cooked onions, garlic and cooking liquid from the casserole into a clean pan and use a hand blender to blitz the mixture to a smooth gravy. If it is too thick, let it down with a splash of hot water. If it's watery, reduce over a medium heat until you achieve the consistency of gravy (it should coat the back of a spoon).

To serve, drain the pickled red onions made at the start, discarding the vinegar. Stir in the mint and parsley. Slice the pork into 5 glorious pieces and serve with the thick onion gravy and pickled red onions.

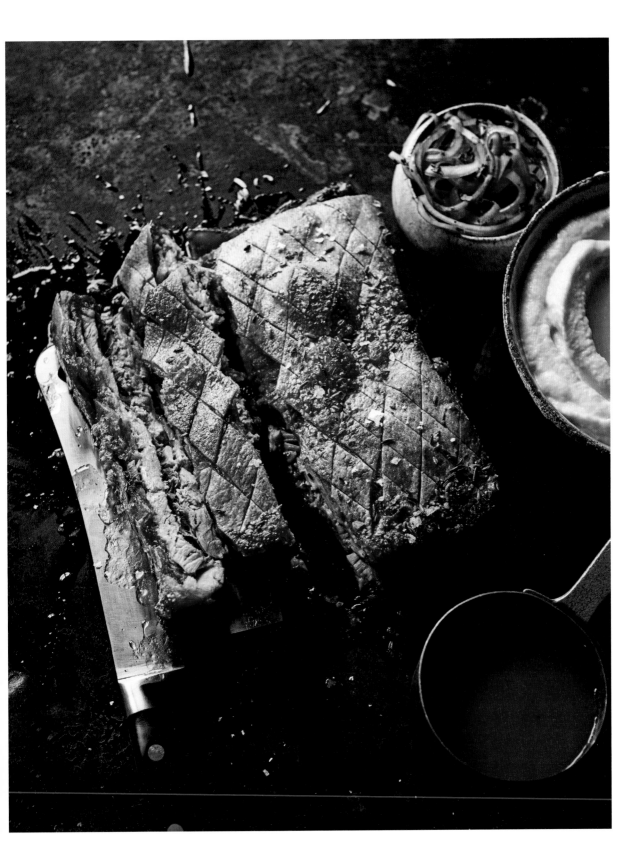

Mustard Pork Chops

with Kale & Celeriac

This tasty, uncomplicated dinner option boasts juicy pork chops and roasted celeriac that has been lightly seasoned with sage. I throw in some kale too, which crisps up beautifully and offers plenty of texture with each mouthful. The mustard element is simply Dijon mustard lightly spread onto each chop after cooking, bringing a lovely acidity to the dish. The roasted celeriac offers just the right amount of sweetness and will have you forgetting all about the apples often enjoyed with pork.

4 SERVINGS   **25m** PREP TIME   **30m** COOK TIME

CALORIES 734 | CARBOHYDRATES 4.4G | PROTEIN 45G | FAT 58G

1 small–medium celeriac (see Tip)

4 teaspoons lard

1 teaspoon dried sage, plus an extra pinch

4 large pork chops (approx. 240g/8½oz each)

70g (2½oz) curly kale, torn

salt flakes, salt and freshly ground black pepper

2 tablespoons Dijon mustard, to serve

The celeriac I used was 670g (1lb 8oz). The macros have been calculated on its trimmed weight, which was 500g (1lb 2oz).

Preheat the oven to 220°C/200°C fan/425°F/gas mark 7.

Trim and peel the celeriac using a good-quality peeler. Wipe the celeriac clean, then dice into 2cm (¾in) pieces. Set aside in a bowl.

Melt 2 teaspoons of the lard, then pour it over the diced celeriac. Add the 1 teaspoon of dried sage and toss well to evenly coat. Spread out on a large roasting tray and bake in the oven for 20–25 minutes.

While the celeriac is cooking, remove the pork chops from their packaging. Pat dry with kitchen paper and season all sides with salt.

Melt the remaining 2 teaspoons of lard in a frying pan over a high heat and fry the pork chops by standing them up on their fatty ends to render and crisp the fat, then frying on their sides until golden and crispy. Scatter over a pinch of dried sage and season with freshly ground black pepper. Set aside to keep warm.

Have the kale prepped and ready in a bowl. Pour the fat and juices from the frying pan you cooked the pork chops in over the kale and use your hands to rub in the juices and evenly coat the kale. Season with salt.

Remove the celeriac from the oven and test a piece – it should be completely cooked through. Add the kale to the tray and return to the oven for 3–4 minutes for the kale to crisp up.

Season the whole lot with salt flakes. Serve the pork with the kale and celeriac – and don't forget to spread a little Dijon mustard over each pork chop just before tucking in!

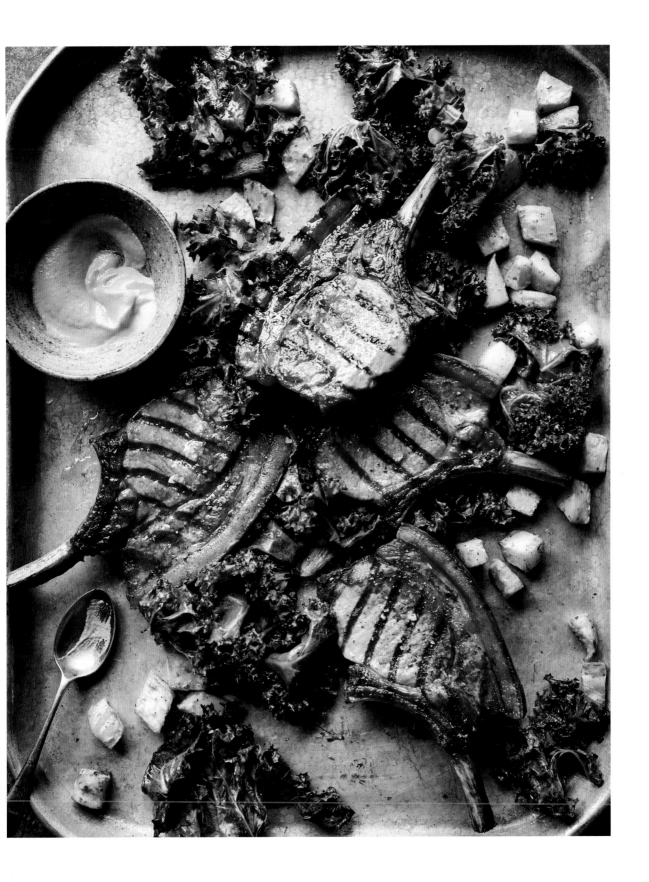

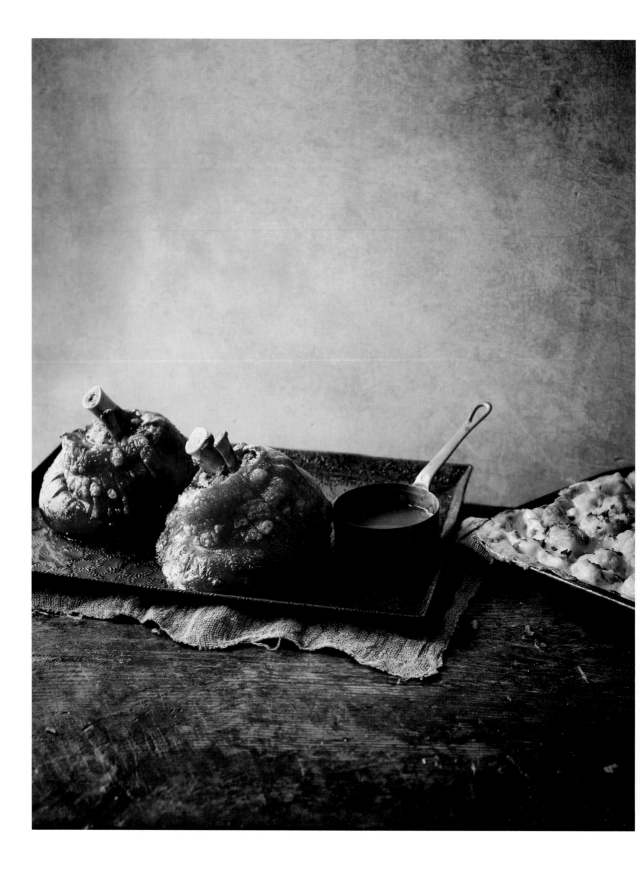

Pork Shanks
with Mustard Gravy

6 SERVINGS

10m PREP TIME

4¼hrs COOK TIME

This is perfect for lazy Sundays in winter! I source fresh pork shanks from my butcher (ask them to score the fat for you) and slow-cook them in a casserole along with onions, garlic and stock. A thick, flavourful gravy is made from the cooked-down onions, fat and juices, which I then enhance with acidic mustard, really making the dish sing. Two shanks will satisfy a party of six, when enjoyed with lovely side vegetables, but if you decide to only cook one shank, follow the recipe and freeze any unused gravy.

CALORIES 658 | CARBOHYDRATES 4.9G | PROTEIN 39G | FAT 53G

2 large onions, very thinly sliced

3 garlic cloves, very thinly sliced

500ml (18fl oz) warm best-quality beef stock

2 fresh (not cured) pork shanks (approx. 1.2kg/2lb 10oz each)

1 tablespoon Dijon mustard

salt and freshly ground black pepper

Preheat the oven to 180°C/160°C fan/350°F/gas mark 4.

Place the onions and garlic into a deep roasting casserole dish (one that has a well-fitting lid) and pour in the beef stock. Season the shanks with salt and black pepper and place in the casserole dish.

Cover the dish with the lid and cook in the oven for 2 hours.

Add 250ml (9fl oz) hot water, being careful not to splash the skin of the shanks too much. Return to the oven, covered, for another hour.

Check the mixture and add a dash of hot water to ensure the onions do not burn. Cook for 1 more hour.

After the full 4 hours, remove the casserole from the oven. Gently remove the shanks and place onto a clean, shallow roasting dish. Crank up the oven temperature to maximum and return the shanks to the oven, uncovered, for approximately 10–15 minutes, to allow the skin to puff up and crisp.

Tip the onions, garlic and stock juices from the casserole dish into a small pan. Use a hand blender to blitz the mixture well. You will notice that the onions, as well as all the rendered fat emulsifying into the stock, will turn the sauce a light, creamy colour once you start blitzing. If it is too thick, let it down with a splash of water. If it is too watery, reduce it over a medium heat, whisking occasionally. The gravy will become darker and thicker as it reduces. It should be thick enough to coat the back of a spoon. Whisk in the Dijon mustard to finish.

To serve, slide away the crispy, puffed crackling from the shanks and serve it alongside the meat, which should easily come off the bones. Enjoy with the delicious gravy and your favourite side dish.

The emulsification of the rendered pork fat and beef stock will make your gravy thick and glossy. It needs to be made just before serving as the fat may split if left standing too long.

Barbecue Lamb Cutlets

with Rosemary Butter

 6 SERVINGS

 10m PREP TIME

 20m COOK TIME

 1hr+ FIRMING TIME

Hands down, lamb is my favourite red meat. Those who love it as much as I do will be aware that lamb and rosemary complement each other very well, so this inspired me to make a quick flavoured butter to pimp my barbecued cutlets. Flavouring butter with herbs or spices is a fantastic way to create interesting dishes, so let the method in this recipe inspire you. For example, you could make a dill butter to melt over grilled fish or drizzle a truffle butter over your rib-eye. Serve with a lovely green salad on the side or any other vegetables that take your fancy.

CALORIES 607 | CARBOHYDRATES 0.5G | PROTEIN 41G | FAT 49G

3 fresh rosemary sprigs

75g (2¾oz) unsalted butter, softened

2 garlic cloves, minced

12 lamb cutlets (approx. 110g/3¾oz each)

salt flakes, salt and freshly ground black pepper

Start with the rosemary butter. Remove the leaves from the rosemary stalks and chop them very finely.

Place the softened butter (which is simply butter left at room temperature for a few hours) in a small bowl and tip in the finely chopped rosemary. Add the minced garlic (using a garlic crusher is best for this recipe) and season with a generous pinch of salt. Combine well before tipping the mixture out onto a piece of clingfilm.

Roll the butter in the clingfilm to form an even 'log', approximately 3cm (1¼in) in diameter (you will be slicing this into 12 discs later, so bear this in mind). Twist the ends of the clingfilm and place in the refrigerator to set for at least an hour until firm.

To cook, prepare your barbecue. Once the coals are ready, cook the lamb as you normally would, turning occasionally until the fat has crisped, and the cutlets are done to your liking.

Just before removing them from the barbecue, remove the log of butter from the refrigerator, unwrap the clingfilm and slice into 12 even-sized discs. Place a disc of butter on each cutlet and allow to melt.

Season with salt flakes and freshly ground black pepper before serving.

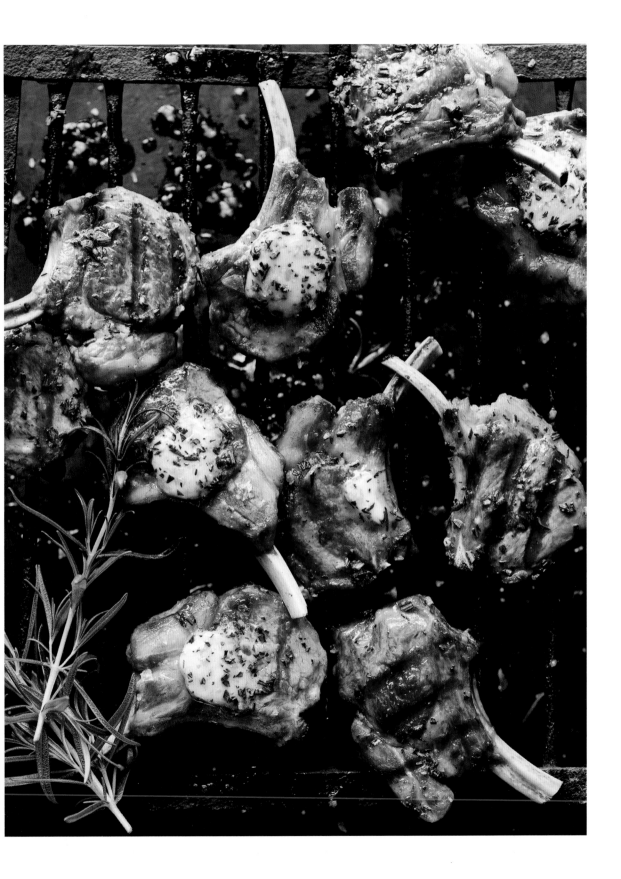

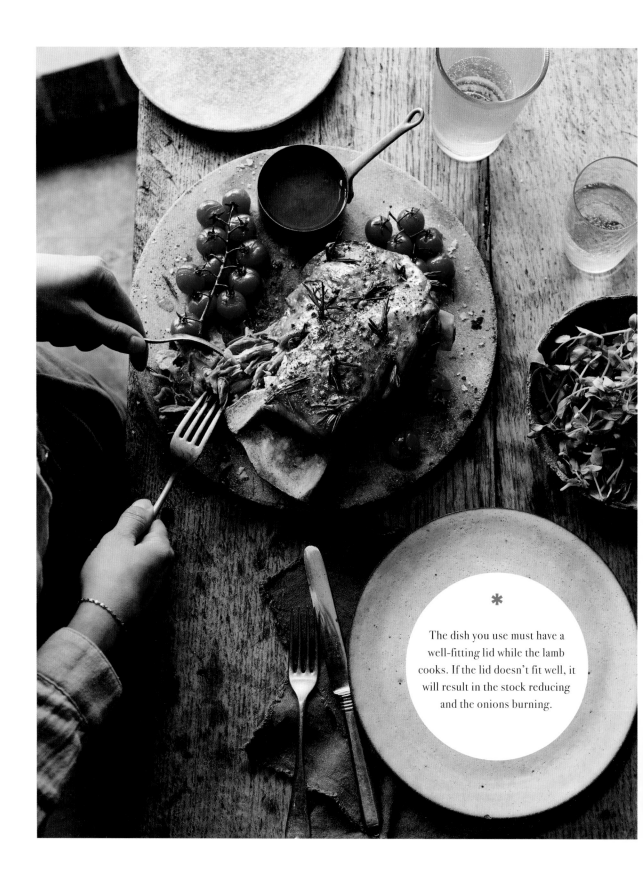

*

The dish you use must have a
well-fitting lid while the lamb
cooks. If the lid doesn't fit well, it
will result in the stock reducing
and the onions burning.

Slow-cooked Lamb Shoulder

with Roasted Cherry Tomatoes

This is an easy recipe for a beautiful slow-cooked lamb shoulder that slides off the bone. The key is three hours of cooking low and slow. The quick-roasted cherry tomatoes add a lovely sweet bite with every mouthful. The flesh from a 1.5kg (3lb 5oz) lamb shoulder (after cooking and removing the bone) will sufficiently feed six people – remember that I also incorporate all the rendered fat from the shoulder into the gravy, making the dish incredibly rich. I love serving it on lazy Sundays with my Cauliflower Cheese Bake (page 110) and greens.

6 SERVINGS | **15m** PREP TIME | **3¼hrs** COOK TIME

CALORIES 551 | CARBOHYDRATES 7.8G | PROTEIN 38G | FAT 40G

For the lamb

2 onions, very thinly sliced

4 garlic cloves, very thinly sliced

500ml (18fl oz) warm best-quality beef stock

lamb shoulder, on the bone (approx. 1.5kg/3lb 5oz)

several fresh rosemary sprigs

several fresh thyme sprigs

1 tablespoon olive oil

salt and freshly ground black pepper

For the tomatoes

360g (12½oz) cherry tomatoes

1 teaspoon olive oil

pinch of salt

The emulsification of the rendered lamb fat and gelatinous beef stock will make your gravy thick and glossy. It needs to be made just before serving as the fat may separate if left standing too long.

Preheat the oven to 180°C/160°C fan/350°F/gas mark 4.

Place the onions and half of the garlic into a deep roasting dish or casserole with a well-fitting lid and pour in the beef stock.

Make small, deep, evenly spaced incisions around all sides of the lamb. Insert the remaining garlic slices into these incisions, along with little snipped pieces of rosemary and thyme. Rub the olive oil all over the lamb and season. Place the lamb into the casserole on top of the onions and garlic. If you have any herbs left over, pop them into the stock too.

Cover with the lid and place in the oven for 3 hours. Check on it every hour and spoon some of the juice over the lamb.

Remove from the oven and gently place the lamb on a serving dish. Remove and discard any of the herbs sticking out from the incisions – they have done their job. Cover the lamb and set aside to keep warm.

Pick out and discard any herbs you see in the onion mixture in the casserole. Tip the entire mixture into a small pan and use a hand blender to blitz well. The onions, as well as all the rendered fat emulsifying into the stock, will turn the sauce a light, creamy colour. Once completely emulsified, heat the mixture over a low–medium heat, whisking occasionally. The gravy will darken and thicken as it reduces.

Meanwhile, crank the oven temperature up to maximum. Spread the tomatoes out on a tray and drizzle over the olive oil. Season with a pinch of salt and roast for 5–7 minutes until the skins start to burst.

Once ready to eat, slide the rested meat from the bones and use 2 forks to break up the lovely soft lamb flesh. Serve with the gravy and sweet roasted tomatoes.

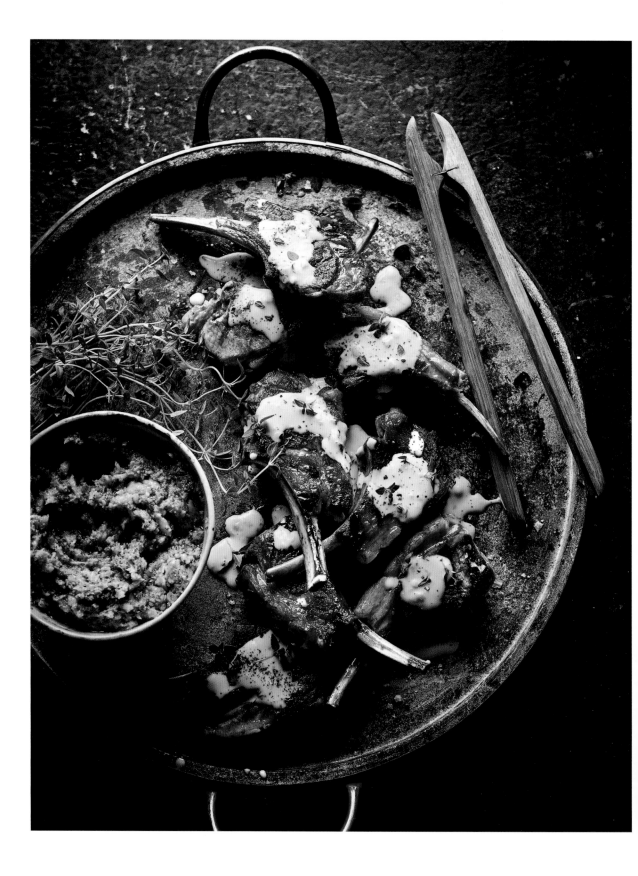

Lamb Cutlets
with a Creamy Garlic Thyme Sauce

These grilled lamb cutlets are finished in a dreamy garlic and thyme sauce and are extraordinarily tasty! Serve with your choice of side vegetables, like Browned Butter Broccoli Mash, as pictured (page 110), or Asparagus with Parmesan (page 111).

4 SERVINGS | **15m** PREP TIME | **20m** COOK TIME

CALORIES 677 | CARBOHYDRATES 1.6G | PROTEIN 36G | FAT 58G

8 lamb cutlets (approx. 110g/3¾oz each)

5g (⅛oz) lard

3 garlic cloves, crushed

2 tablespoons picked fresh thyme leaves (see Tip)

60ml (4 tablespoons) dry white wine

170ml (5¾fl oz) double cream

salt flakes, salt and freshly ground black pepper

Remove the lamb cutlets from their packaging and pat dry with kitchen paper. Season both sides with a little salt and black pepper.

The lamb can either be grilled on the *braai* (barbecue) or on the hob. Just get some good colour on both sides without overcooking them. I advise grilling the fat end first to render and crisp that glorious strip of heaven, before cooking the cutlets on their sides. This may involve some careful balancing of the cutlets side by side on their fatty side, but it's worth it.

While the lamb is cooking, prepare the accompanying sauce. Melt the lard in a large, non-stick pan over a low heat and lightly fry the crushed garlic. Add the thyme leaves, followed by the white wine and cook until all the wine has evaporated and cooked out. Pour in the cream and cook for 3–4 minutes over a medium heat until the cream reduces to a thick sauce.

When the cutlets are done, spoon over the sauce and season the lamb with salt flakes to serve.

Picking thyme leaves is notoriously mind-numbing. Running your fingers along each sprig removes the leaves efficiently. You'll need a generous handful of thyme sprigs to yield two tablespoons.

Simple Roasted Bone Marrow

2 SERVINGS · 5m PREP TIME · 25m COOK TIME

Be still, my heart; it's bone marrow! Marrow needs nothing else other than to be roasted well, then seasoned. I scoop mine out and spread it on slices of toasted Mixed Seed Bread Loaf (page 20), but don't forget that it requires a generous scattering of salt flakes and fresh herbs.

(EXCLUDING BREAD) CALORIES 569 | CARBOHYDRATES 0.5G | PROTEIN 1.3G | FAT 62G

4 bone marrow troughs (approx. 170g/6oz each)

generous pinch of salt flakes

fresh herbs of your choice

Preheat the oven to 220°C/200°C fan/425°F/gas mark 7.

Open the packaging and remove the bone marrow pieces. Pat dry with kitchen paper and place, cut side-up, on a roasting tray. Roast in the oven for 25 minutes.

Season with salt flakes and scatter over the herbs of your choice. Scoop out the gloriously fatty marrow and spread onto slices of toasted Mixed Seed Bread Loaf (which can be toasted by simply frying in a little butter on both sides until golden).

Calves' Liver
with Creamed Cabbage

2 SERVINGS · 15m PREP TIME · 15m COOK TIME

Liver is one of most nutrient-dense foods you can eat and it's highly recommended that you include it in your diet. If you can't source calves' liver, lambs' liver is a suitable alternative. If liver isn't to your liking, try the creamed cabbage as a side dish. *Pictured on page 109, bottom right.*

CALORIES 594 | CARBOHYDRATES 7.1G | PROTEIN 30G | FAT 49G

For the creamed cabbage

10g (¼oz) unsalted butter

100g (3½oz) smoked bacon lardons

2 garlic cloves thinly sliced

160g (5¾oz) Savoy cabbage (inner leaves), very thinly sliced

50ml (1¾fl oz) dry white wine

100ml (3½fl oz) double cream

freshly ground black pepper

For the liver

200g (7oz) sliced calves' liver

2 teaspoons lard

1 tablespoon fresh thyme leaves, to serve

salt flakes

Melt the butter in a large, non-stick pan over a medium heat and add the bacon and garlic. Cook until the bacon cooks through and releases all its fat and juices. Add the cabbage and white wine and stir until the cabbage completely wilts and the white wine evaporates and cooks out. Add the double cream to warm through and reduce to thicken.

The bacon will provide plenty of saltiness, so a generous crack of ground black pepper is all that is needed. Set aside to keep warm.

Remove the liver from its packaging and drain in a colander if needed. Pat the pieces dry with kitchen paper. Melt the lard in a non-stick pan over a very high heat. Once smoking hot, sear the pieces on all sides until browned (this doesn't take long and you don't want to overcook the liver). Season with salt flakes and freshly ground black pepper.

Serve the liver on top of the cabbage and scatter over fresh thyme leaves before serving.

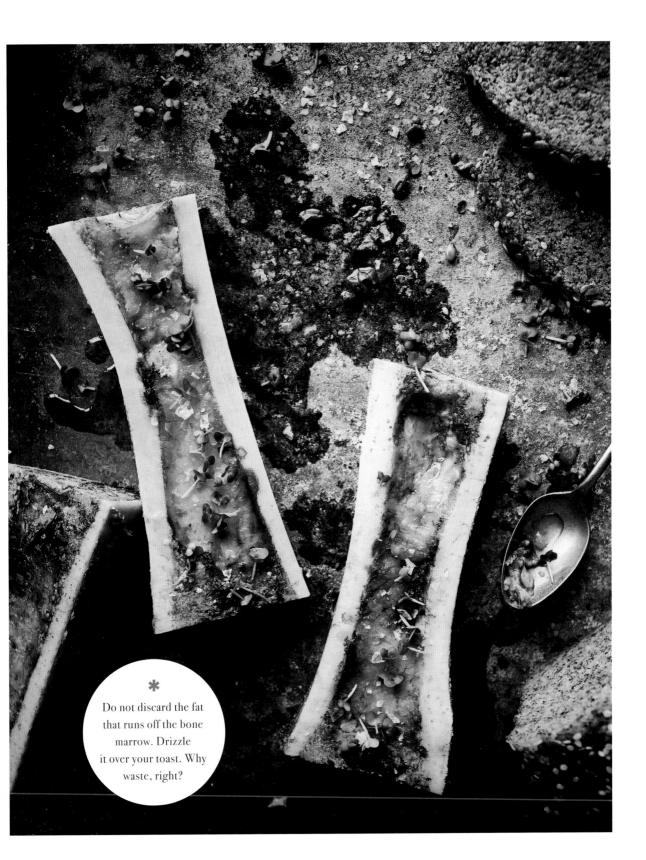

*

Do not discard the fat
that runs off the bone
marrow. Drizzle
it over your toast. Why
waste, right?

Spicy Chicken Livers

Many people aren't entirely convinced about how delightful chicken livers are. I think it's possibly the texture of over-cooked livers, which tend to be crumbly. I have offered a method here to get them cooked just right. The homemade spicy sauce can be made ahead of time, but it does take some patience. Don't be discouraged, the results are worth it! When prepping your chicken livers, drain them very well in a colander before removing the sinew and stringy bits. Chop them into smaller pieces to ensure even cooking.

4 SERVINGS | **20m** PREP TIME | **1¼hrs** COOK TIME

CALORIES 404 | CARBOHYDRATES 9.2G | PROTEIN 27G | FAT 28G

40g (1½oz) unsalted butter

400g (14oz) chicken livers, chopped small (trimmed weight)

170g (6oz) mushrooms, quartered

1 tablespoon red wine vinegar

65g (2½oz) soured cream

salt flakes, salt and freshly ground black pepper

small handful of fresh flat-leaf parsley, finely chopped, to serve

For the spicy sauce

400g (14oz) chopped tomatoes, canned or fresh

1 small red onion, roughly chopped

1 small red pepper, roughly chopped

3 garlic cloves, roughly chopped

1 large red chilli, seeds removed and roughly chopped, plus extra to serve (optional)

1 tablespoon red wine vinegar

1 lemon, peeled, flesh segments only, pips removed

Begin with the spicy sauce. Simply place all the ingredients into a mini food processor/food chopper and blitz well. Tip the mixture into a medium-sized non-stick pan and cook over a low–medium heat for 40–45 minutes, stirring occasionally. Blitz the cooked mixture a second time. Set aside until needed.

For the livers, melt half the butter in a large non-stick pan over a high heat. Add the livers and cook until they brown and caramelize on the outside. They will soon release their own moisture, so allow this to evaporate. (You may need to cook the liver in 2 batches.) Remove the browned livers and set them aside on a plate. Season with a little salt.

Using the same pan, add the remaining butter along with the mushrooms and reduce the heat to medium. The mushrooms will immediately soak up all the butter. Add the red wine vinegar to deglaze, using your spatula or wooden spoon to scrape any pieces stuck to the bottom.

Tip in the spicy sauce along with 60ml (4 tablespoons) hot water. Give the mixture a good stir and return the livers to the pan. Cook for approximately 7–8 minutes until the sauce thickens and the livers cook through a little more.

The jury is out on whether chicken livers can safely be enjoyed while still slightly pink on the inside, but I love them this way. If you prefer them cooked more, simply keep them on the heat a little longer – but please avoid overcooking them, as their texture will change.

To serve, stir through the soured cream and season with salt flakes and freshly ground black pepper. Scatter over the finely chopped parsley and additional sliced red chilli if you are feeling brave!

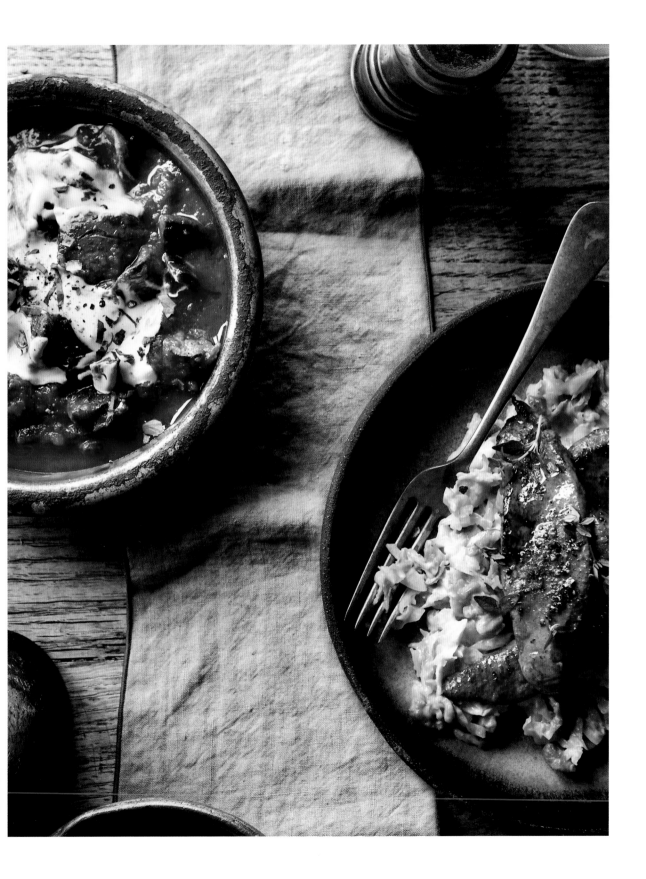

Browned Butter Broccoli Mash

 4 SERVINGS AS A SIDE

 10m PREP TIME

 25m COOK TIME

400g (14oz) broccoli florets

90g (3¼oz) unsalted butter

2 garlic cloves, thinly sliced

salt, salt flakes

I love broccoli in all forms, but really wanted to showcase this version where I mashed it in a browned butter infused with garlic. It may not seem like a generous side dish, but the richness and flavour of it go a long way on your plate. *Pictured on page 104.*

CALORIES 193 | CARBOHYDRATES 3.2G | PROTEIN 4.3G | FAT 18G

Bring a pan of salted water to the boil. Add the broccoli and cook for 15–18 minutes until the florets have completely softened. Drain well and allow the moisture to steam off. Return the broccoli to a clean, dry pan (or just wipe the one you used) and mash very well using a potato masher.

Melt the butter in a small pan over a medium heat. Once it starts to foam, add the garlic and swirl the pan. The butter will start browning. Remove from the heat and allow to infuse for 5 minutes.

Line a sieve with muslin or cheesecloth and strain the butter into the mashed broccoli. Discard the contents of the muslin. Mix the mash to combine. Warm through and season with salt flakes before serving.

Cauliflower Cheese Bake

 6 SERVINGS AS A SIDE

 10m PREP TIME

 50m COOK TIME

750g (1lb 10oz) cauliflower florets, trimmed into small, equal-sized pieces

420ml (15fl oz) double cream

generous pinch of ground nutmeg

3 garlic cloves, smashed with the back of a knife

100g (3½oz) extra-mature full-fat Cheddar cheese, grated

small handful of fresh flat-leaf parsley, finely chopped, to serve

salt and ground white pepper

salt flakes and freshly ground black pepper

I am so pleased to share this easy recipe with you to enjoy as a side veg option to your Sunday roast. The flavour of baked cream is luxurious and satisfying and does a fantastic job of mimicking the white sauce we associate with a baked cauliflower cheese. *Pictured on page 98.*

CALORIES 444 | CARBOHYDRATES 4.9G | PROTEIN 9.8G | FAT 42G

Preheat the oven to 200°C/180°C fan/400°F/gas mark 6.

Bring a large pan of salted water to the boil and add the cauliflower. Boil for 15–18 minutes until softened. Drain and transfer to a suitably sized baking dish and season with salt flakes and black pepper.

Meanwhile, heat the double cream in a pan over a low heat. Add the nutmeg and smashed garlic. Season with salt and white pepper and simmer for a minute or two. Strain through a sieve (discarding the smashed garlic) and pour over the cauliflower. Bake for 20 minutes.

Remove from the oven and increase the temperature to 220°C/200°C fan/425°F/gas mark 7. Scatter over the grated cheese and return to the hotter oven for 15 minutes until the cheese bubbles and gratins. Season and scatter over chopped parsley before serving.

Asparagus
with Parmesan

Great vegetables need very little to make them shine. Use the largest, fattest fresh asparagus you can find as it makes shaving the ends off a lot easier. If you cannot source Parmesan, use Pecorino, Grana Padano, Pecorino Romano or Parmigiano-Reggiano. *Pictured on page 61.*

4 SERVINGS AS A SIDE   **15m** PREP TIME   **5m** COOK TIME

CALORIES 117 | CARBOHYDRATES 1.6G | PROTEIN 4G | FAT 10G

500g (1lb 2oz) large asparagus, woody ends removed and bottom half shaved with a peeler (see Tip)

40g (1½oz) unsalted butter

20g (¾oz) Parmesan, finely grated

salt

Snapping off the woody ends and shaving off the bottom half makes the asparagus look more beautiful and green, and makes the texture less stringy.

Bring a wide-bottomed pan of salted water to the boil. Add the asparagus and boil for 2–4 minutes, depending on their thickness. You don't want to over-cook them as they will lose their beautiful colour.

Remove the asparagus from the water and place on a plate lined with kitchen paper to drain. Season well with salt. Place onto a serving platter and set aside to keep warm.

Add the butter to a clean pan over a medium heat and allow it to melt and foam. As soon as it stops sizzling, remove the pan from the heat and pour the butter over the warm asparagus. Scatter with the Parmesan and serve immediately.

Creamed Spinach

Not to sound boastful, but I truly believe this will be the best creamed spinach you will ever eat. From start to finish, you are 20 minutes away from your new favourite side dish! *Pictured on page 112.*

4 SERVINGS AS A SIDE   **10m** PREP TIME   **10m** COOK TIME

CALORIES 174 | CARBOHYDRATES 1.6G | PROTEIN 4.2G | FAT 17G

2 teaspoons unsalted butter

500g (1lb 2oz) baby spinach leaves

1 teaspoon garlic powder

80ml (2¾fl oz) double cream

80g (2¾oz) soured cream

salt and ground white pepper

Melt the butter in a large non-stick pan over a medium heat. Add half the spinach to the pan and stir continuously until the leaves wilt. This will leave you with enough space to add the remaining spinach.

Cook until all the spinach has completely wilted down. Use a spatula to chop/mash the mixture to a pulp as you stir it around the pan. Add the garlic powder, cooking for a few seconds, before adding the cream and soured cream. Season with salt and white pepper and continue to cook over a medium heat until both creams thicken and you are left with a thick, creamy spinach mixture. Heaven!

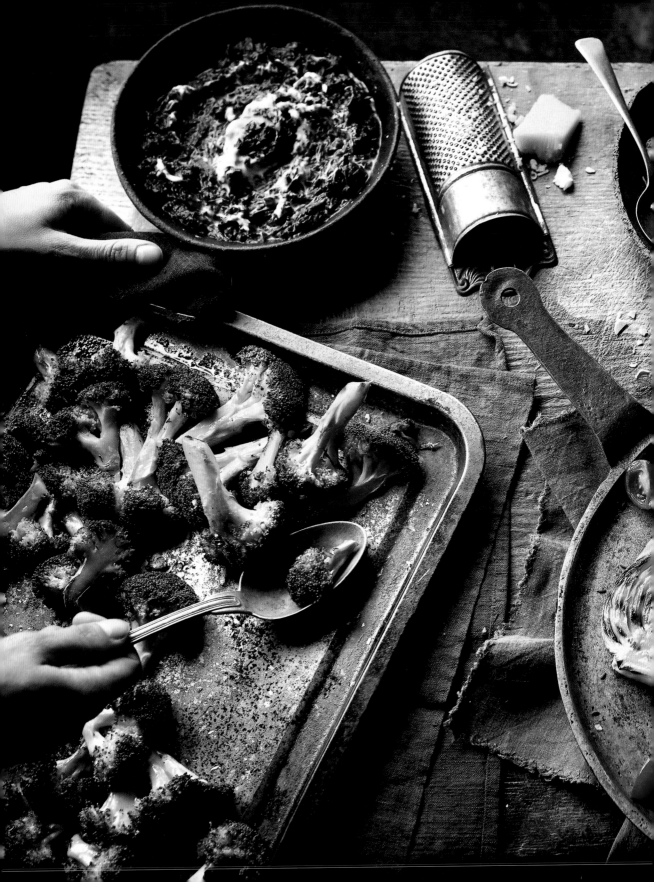

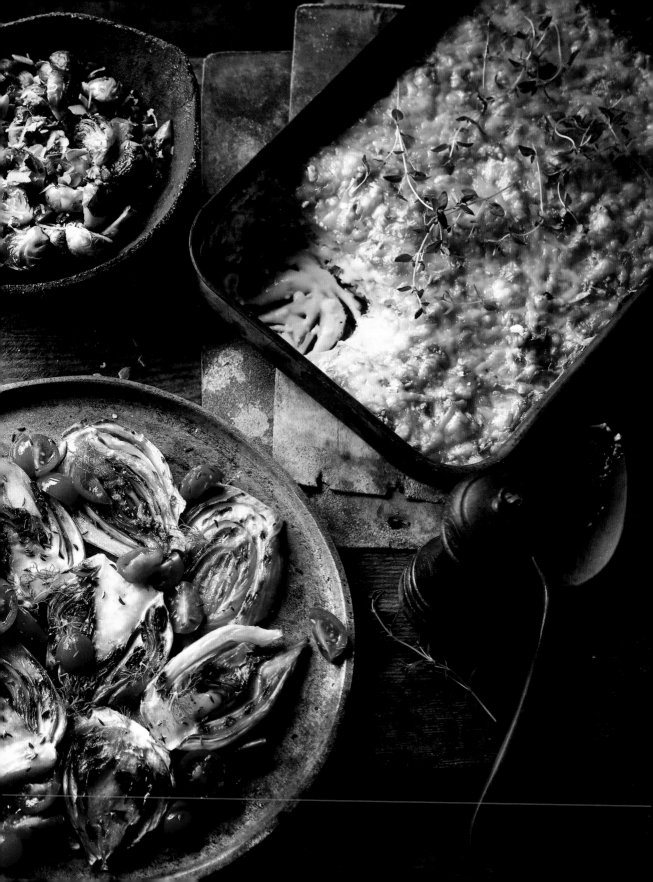

Celeriac Dauphinoise

6–8 SERVINGS AS A SIDE | **20m** PREP TIME | **1hr 10** COOK TIME

The keto police may steer you far away from root vegetables, but celeriac is low enough in carbs if the amounts are monitored! It is also a fantastic substitute for potatoes and boasts a lovely flavour. I based the macros on a generous 175g (6oz) serving per person. *Pictured on page 113.*

CALORIES 533 | CARBOHYDRATES 4.2G | PROTEIN 6.6G | FAT 53G

20g (¾oz) unsalted butter

4 garlic cloves, very thinly sliced

600ml (20fl oz) double cream

2 small–medium celeriac, trimmed, peeled and thinly sliced with a mandolin (my celeriac had a combined total weight of 1.35kg (3lb), and their trimmed weight was 900g (2lb).

100g (3½oz) Gruyère cheese, grated

salt and ground white pepper

salt flakes and fresh thyme, to serve

Preheat the oven to 170°/150°C fan/340°F/gas mark 3½.

Melt the butter in a pan over a low heat and gently cook the garlic until softened. Add the cream and season. Warm through, then set aside.

Layer the celeriac in a large roasting dish, ladling in a little warm cream between each layer. Cover tightly with foil and bake for 30 minutes.

Reduce the oven temperature to 160°C/140°C fan/325°F/gas mark 3 and remove the foil. Use a spatula to compress the celeriac slices down into the baking cream. Scatter over the Gruyère cheese and return the dish, uncovered, to the oven for another 30 minutes. Season with sea salt flakes and scatter over the thyme leaves before tucking in!

Best-ever Roasted Brussels Sprouts

4 SERVINGS AS A SIDE | **10m** PREP TIME | **25m** COOK TIME

As a child I used to hide Brussels sprouts under my napkin. I am so glad I outgrew that crazy thinking because I love them now ! Enjoy this with a Sunday roast, or as a side dish option to your midweek grilled chicken or steak. *Pictured on page 113.*

CALORIES 263 | CARBOHYDRATES 4.9G | PROTEIN 14G | FAT 20G

15g (½oz) flaked almonds

2 tablespoons unsalted butter

200g (7oz) smoked bacon lardons

400g (14oz) Brussels sprouts, trimmed and halved

½ teaspoon garlic powder

20g (¾oz) Parmesan, finely grated, to serve

freshly ground black pepper

Preheat the oven to 200°C/180°C fan/400°F/gas mark 6.

Toast the flaked almonds in a dry frying pan over a medium heat until golden. Remove and crush lightly using a pestle and mortar. Set aside.

Add the butter and bacon lardons to the same pan and cook over a medium heat until the bacon cooks through and releases all its fat and juices. Pour the bacon – including the fat and juices – into a bowl with the Brussels sprouts. Add the garlic powder and mix well to combine.

Spread out on a large baking tray and roast for 15–20 minutes. To serve, scatter over the crushed almonds and grated Parmesan and finish with a crack of black pepper.

Fennel
with Caraway & Tomatoes

Adding toasted caraway and sweet tomatoes to fennel gives an interesting flavour dimension. I recommend you enjoy this side veg option alongside simple lamb chops or grilled chicken to avoid any competing flavours. *Pictured on page 113.*

 4 SERVINGS AS A SIDE **5m** PREP TIME **15m** COOK TIME

CALORIES 61 | CARBOHYDRATES 3G | PROTEIN 1.4G | FAT 4.2G

2 teaspoons caraway seeds

1 tablespoon lard

2 fennel bulbs, cut into 1.5cm (⅝in) slices lengthways (retain the fronds for garnish)

250ml (9fl oz) vegetable stock

2 teaspoons white wine vinegar

60g (2¼oz) cherry tomatoes, halved

Toast the caraway seeds in a large, dry, non-stick pan over a medium heat. Once they begin to colour, remove from the pan and set aside.

Melt the lard in the same pan and add the sliced fennel. Cook on all sides over a high heat until golden and caramelized. Pour in the vegetable stock and white wine vinegar and reduce the heat to medium. Return the toasted caraway seeds to the pan.

Keep the pan on the heat until all the vegetable stock evaporates, adding the halved tomatoes in the last minute of cooking. This will be enough time for the fennel to cook through without losing its shape. Garnish with fennel fronds before serving.

Coconut-roasted Broccoli

This is the perfect side dish to enjoy on keto. Don't just use broccoli florets – the stems are delicious and should be included too. They soften and melt in your mouth while the florets caramelize and crisp up; it's a beautiful texture combination. *Pictured on page 112.*

 4 SERVINGS AS A SIDE **5m** PREP TIME **25m** COOK TIME

CALORIES 179 | CARBOHYDRATES 4.4G | PROTEIN 5.9G | FAT 15G

550g (1lb 4oz) broccoli (approximately 1 large head)

55g (2oz) coconut oil

salt flakes

Preheat the oven to 200°C/180°C fan/400°F/gas mark 6.

Trim the broccoli into evenly sized, chunky pieces. This is best done by halving each floret. Do not discard the stems, they are delicious. Place into a large bowl.

Place the coconut oil in a suitable bowl and heat in the microwave on medium for 20 seconds until completely melted. Pour the coconut oil over the broccoli and toss well to evenly coat. Spread the broccoli out on a large roasting tray. Roast in the oven for 25 minutes until the stems have softened and the ends of the florets are golden.

Serve immediately, scattered with salt flakes.

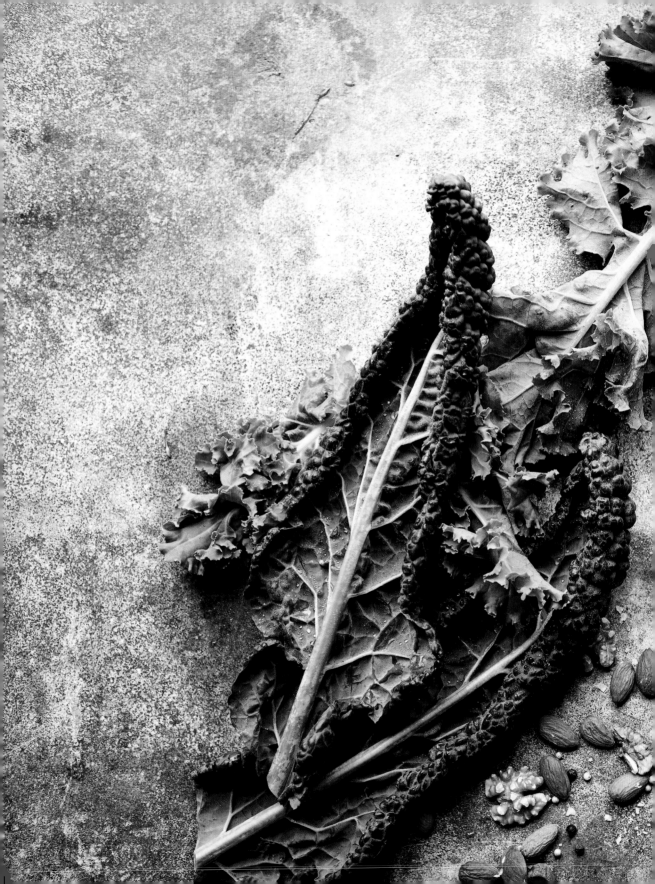

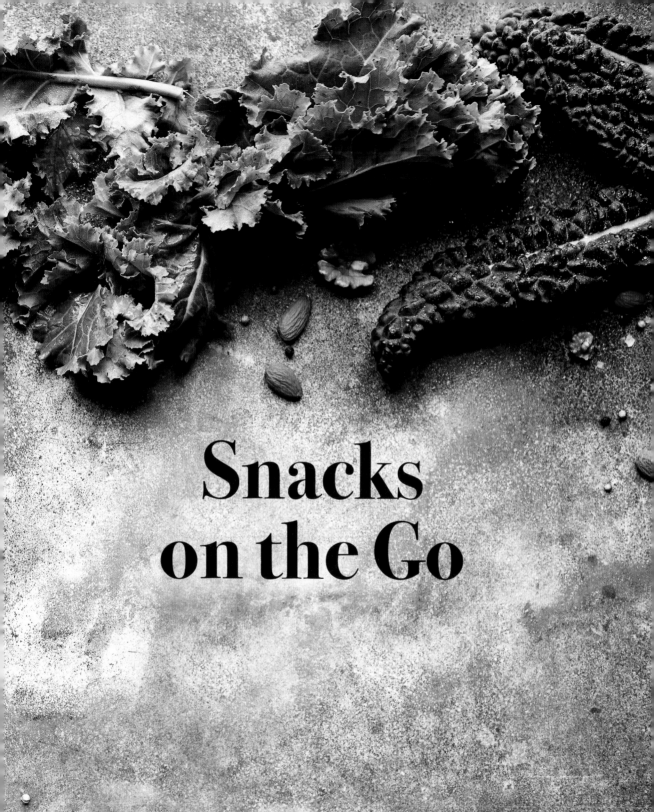

Snacks
on the Go

Cheesy Kale Crisps

2 SERVINGS | **10m** PREP TIME | **5m** COOK TIME

These cheesy kale crisps will make you forget all about the carb-laden snacks while watching the game on Saturdays! They are low in carbs, high in fibre and packed with goodness. Be sure to source whole leaves for this recipe so that you can trim them into even-sized pieces.

CALORIES 156 | CARBOHYDRATES 1.8G | PROTEIN 7.1G | FAT 13G

100g (3½oz) cavolo nero (black kale), trimmed weight (see Tip)

1 tablespoon olive oil

1 tablespoon nutritional yeast flakes

15g (½oz) Parmesan cheese, finely grated

½ teaspoon garlic powder

pinch of ground white pepper

Preheat the oven to 220°C/200°C fan/425°F/gas mark 7.

Trim and discard the large centre stalk from each kale leaf. Chop the leaves into equal-sized pieces, approximately 4cm (1½in), and place in a large bowl. Drizzle over the olive oil and all the remaining ingredients. Get stuck in with your hands to rub the mixture thoroughly into the leaves for even coating.

Spread the kale out on a large roasting tray and cook in the oven for 5 minutes exactly. I have a habit of quickly opening the oven door and rotating the tray halfway through. If you do choose to do this, don't leave the oven door open too long because heat gets lost. Allow the crisps to cool completely before tucking in.

Roasted Macadamia Nuts

7 SERVINGS | **5m** PREP TIME | **12m** COOK TIME

Deeply rich and mind-blowing in flavour, macadamia nuts smell like popcorn and taste like heaven when roasted like this. These high-fat nuts are the ultimate keto snack when you feel the need to crunch on something in between meals. *Pictured on page 120.*

PER 35G (1¼oz SERVING) | CALORIES 273 | CARBOHYDRATES 1.6G | PROTEIN 2.8G | FAT 28G

250g (9oz) macadamia nuts

pinch of salt

pinch of powdered erythritol

Preheat the oven to 200°C/180°C fan/400°F/gas mark 6.

Remove the nuts from the packet in small handfuls and spread out on a tray lined with parchment paper. (I do this because just emptying all the contents from the packet will result in the nut 'dust' that is present at the bottom of the packet being added to the tray – and burning.)

Place the tray into the oven for 10–12 minutes, shaking and rotating halfway through. Remove from the oven and immediately scatter over a pinch of salt and a pinch of erythritol. Toss well to evenly coat.

Allow the nuts to cool completely before storing in a sealed container. They will keep for up to 1 week.

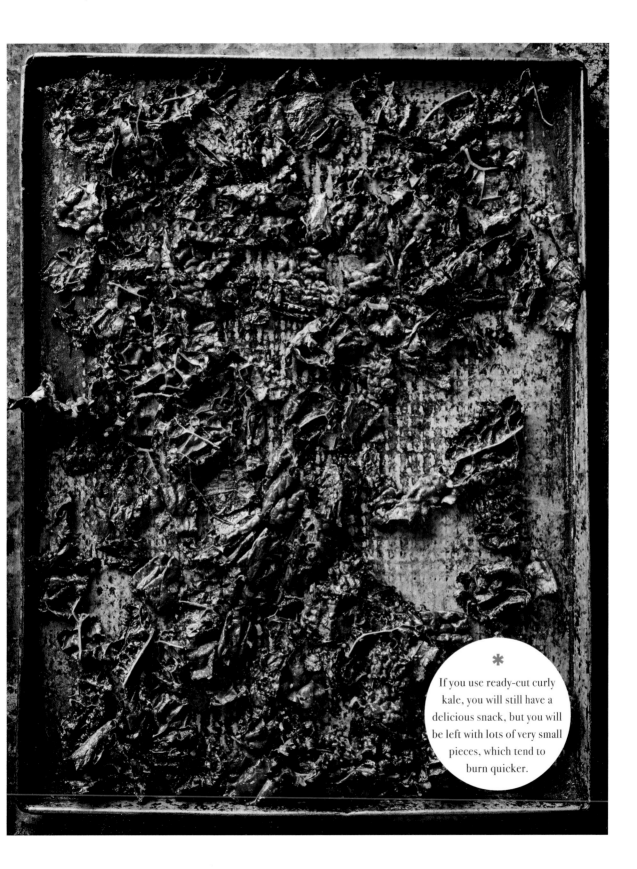

If you use ready-cut curly kale, you will still have a delicious snack, but you will be left with lots of very small pieces, which tend to burn quicker.

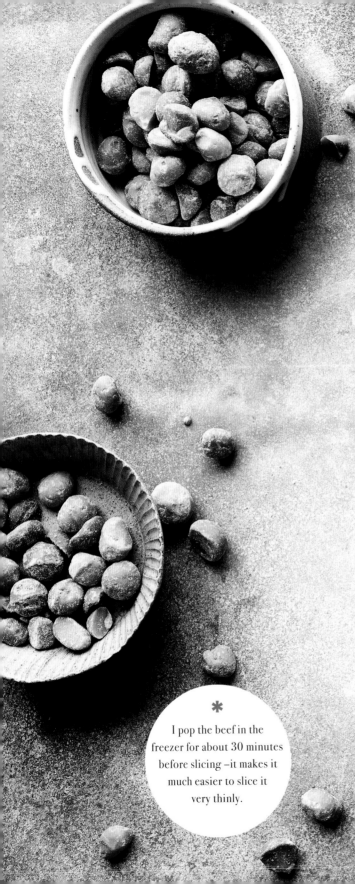

Beef Jerky Two Ways

10–12 SERVINGS

20m PREP TIME

2 hrs COOK TIME

PER 30G (1OZ) SERVING OF SWEET & SPICY JERKY | CALORIES 97 | CARBOHYDRATES 2G | PROTEIN 9.2G | FAT 5.8G |

PER 30G (1OZ) SERVING OF CORIANDER & PEPPER JERKY | CALORIES 91 | CARBOHYDRATES 0G | PROTEIN 9.2G | FAT 5.9G |

I am part proudly South African, and part proudly British, so I had to give a nod to my favourite keto snack ever: cured, dried beef strips!

We call it 'biltong' in South Africa, but it's actually very different to what the rest of the world refers to as 'jerky'. Biltong in South Africa is made by cutting large pieces of beef along the grain, marinating and hanging it to dry, before slicing. I love it fatty and moist, with that quintessential flavour of coriander seeds. Jerky is quite different: it's leaner and often sweeter. Both can be made at home, but the method for jerky is simpler and requires no special equipment. To compromise here, I have offered the method for homemade jerky, but provided two different spice options (and I know which one is my favourite!). The method is the same, whichever spices you choose.

*
I pop the beef in the freezer for about 30 minutes before slicing –it makes it much easier to slice it very thinly.

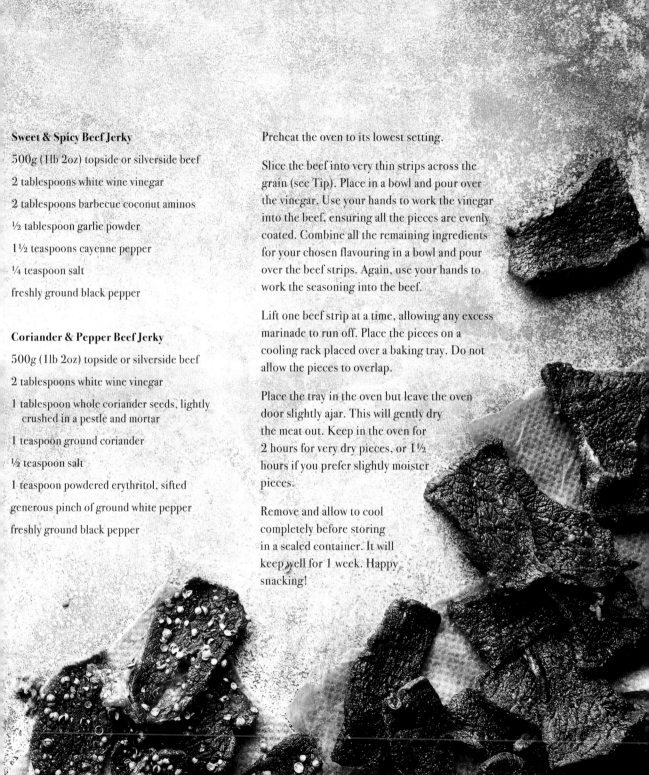

Sweet & Spicy Beef Jerky

500g (1lb 2oz) topside or silverside beef

2 tablespoons white wine vinegar

2 tablespoons barbecue coconut aminos

½ tablespoon garlic powder

1½ teaspoons cayenne pepper

¼ teaspoon salt

freshly ground black pepper

Coriander & Pepper Beef Jerky

500g (1lb 2oz) topside or silverside beef

2 tablespoons white wine vinegar

1 tablespoon whole coriander seeds, lightly
    crushed in a pestle and mortar

1 teaspoon ground coriander

½ teaspoon salt

1 teaspoon powdered erythritol, sifted

generous pinch of ground white pepper

freshly ground black pepper

Preheat the oven to its lowest setting.

Slice the beef into very thin strips across the grain (see Tip). Place in a bowl and pour over the vinegar. Use your hands to work the vinegar into the beef, ensuring all the pieces are evenly coated. Combine all the remaining ingredients for your chosen flavouring in a bowl and pour over the beef strips. Again, use your hands to work the seasoning into the beef.

Lift one beef strip at a time, allowing any excess marinade to run off. Place the pieces on a cooling rack placed over a baking tray. Do not allow the pieces to overlap.

Place the tray in the oven but leave the oven door slightly ajar. This will gently dry the meat out. Keep in the oven for 2 hours for very dry pieces, or 1½ hours if you prefer slightly moister pieces.

Remove and allow to cool completely before storing in a sealed container. It will keep well for 1 week. Happy snacking!

Pork Scratchings

1
BATCH

45m
PREP
TIME

2hr 10
COOK
TIME

1 large sheet of pork skin (ask your butcher)

salt flakes

Hopefully by now you have made good friends with your butcher! Ask him/her for a large sheet of inexpensive pork skin and get cracking at making your own homemade scratchings! The best part of this recipe is that you can change things up. If a simple salt seasoning seems a little dull, add a pinch of smoked paprika or chilli powder to enhance the flavour.

Place the pork skin side-down on a chopping board. Use a very sharp knife to remove as much fat as possible. I recommend wearing food preparation gloves for a better grip on the skin as you slide the fat off. Do this safely by sliding it off away from you.

Pat the sheet dry with kitchen paper and slice into smaller pieces. The size doesn't really matter, but I would advise that each piece is the same width and length as your thumb. Now that you have smaller pieces, you could remove even more fat if you desire. Scatter salt evenly over the pieces and place them on a cooling rack set over a tray. You may need to use 2 trays. In the meantime, preheat the oven to its lowest setting.

Place the tray(s) in the oven for 2 hours. I always keep the oven door slightly ajar, as I want the skins to dry out, not 'cook'.

Remove the tray(s) from the oven and transfer the little pieces onto a clean tray. Crank up the oven temperature to 250°C/230°C fan/500°F/gas mark 9½.

Once the oven is at temperature, return the tray to the oven and cook for 5–7 minutes until you see (and hear) the pieces swell and pop – it's super fun to watch!

Remove the tray from the oven and place the scratchings on a tray lined with kitchen paper. Once cooled, store in a sealed container at room temperature and keep for no longer than a week.

*
I can't provide accurate nutritional information for this recipe as it is too variable. However, the carb count of pork skin will always be 0g.

Cashew & Coconut Fat Bombs

These fat bombs are a perfect grab-and-go option. They should be kept in the refrigerator to hold their shape, but they freeze well too, making them an ideal option for batch-making.

 9 FAT BOMBS

 25m PREP TIME

 15m COOK TIME

 30m FIRMING TIME

PER CASHEW & COCONUT FAT BOMB | CALORIES 170 | CARBOHYDRATES 2.9G | PROTEIN 4.1G | FAT 15G |

PER ALMOND & CINNAMON FAT BOMB | CALORIES 173 | CARBOHYDRATES 1.7G | PROTEIN 4.1G | FAT 16G |

250g (9oz) raw cashew nuts

pinch of salt

60g (2¼oz) almond flour

30g (1oz) coconut flour

35g (1¼oz) powdered erythritol

50g (1¾oz) coconut oil, melted

10g (¼oz) desiccated coconut

 *

Variation: Roasted Almond & Cinnamon Butter Fat Bombs

Follow the same method but replace the coconut flour with extra-fine almond flour, the Cashew Nut Butter with Roasted Almond & Cinnamon Butter (see page 138) and the coconut oil with unflavoured coconut oil. There is no need to roll these in desiccated coconut – they are fabulous as they are!

Preheat the oven to 180°C/160°C fan/350°F/ gas mark 4 and line a baking tray with parchment paper.

Spread the cashew nuts out on the prepared baking tray and bake for 10–12 minutes, shaking and rotating halfway through. Allow to cool slightly, then transfer to a mini food processor with a pinch of salt and blitz well to fine crumbs. Continue to blitz until the mixture starts to look oily and resembles a fairly smooth peanut butter. Weigh out 85g (3oz) to use in these fat bombs and keep the remainder in the refrigerator, covered, for other use. (It will keep for at least 2 weeks – try it spread over a slice of toasted Mixed Seed Bread Loaf (page 20) or stirred into a curry for extra flavour.)

In a separate bowl, combine the almond flour, coconut flour and erythritol. Pour in the melted coconut oil and the 85g (3oz) cashew nut butter. Stir well and chill for 30 minutes so the mixture can solidify and be easier to work with.

Form 9 small balls (approximately 25g/1oz each) from the mixture. Roll each ball in the desiccated coconut and set aside in the refrigerator until ready to enjoy!

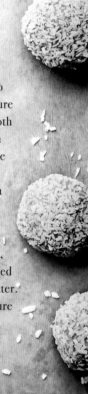

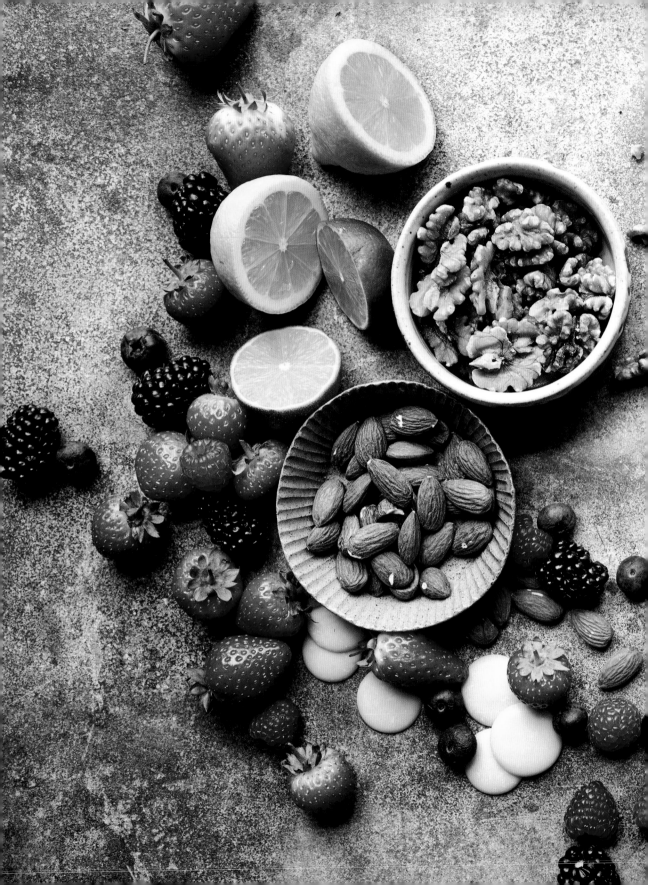

Sweet Treats

Lime Cheesecake

Zingy and creamy, this is a show-stopping dessert that I love to make when I entertain friends. If there are any leftover slices (doubtful), you can store them covered in the refrigerator for a few days or simply wrap them individually and freeze for another day.

 8 SERVINGS   **30m** PREP TIME   **10m** COOK TIME   **5hrs** SETTING TIME

CALORIES 418 | CARBOHYDRATES 4.2G | PROTEIN 6.5G | FAT 41G

For the base

130g (4¾oz) almond flour

2 tablespoons powdered erythritol

45g (1¾oz) unsalted butter, melted

For the cheesecake

4 limes

1½ teaspoons powdered gelatine

300g (10½oz) full-fat cream cheese

40g (1½oz) powdered erythritol, sifted

3–4 drops liquid stevia (optional)

300ml (10fl oz) double cream

To finish

finely grated zest of 1 lime

Preheat the oven to 200°C/180°C fan/400°F/gas mark 6. Grease and line the base and sides of a deep, loose-bottomed tin (20cm/8in diameter) with parchment paper.

Combine the almond flour and erythritol together in a bowl. Pour in the melted butter and combine until the mixture resembles moist breadcrumbs. Tip the mixture into the prepared tin and use your hands to compress it down into an even, compact layer.

Bake for 10 minutes, then remove and allow to cool completely in the tin on a cooling rack.

Use a fine zester to grate the zest of the 4 limes into a bowl. Set aside. Halve each lime and squeeze all the juice into a small pan. Heat this lime juice over a medium heat and scatter in the powdered gelatine. Once the gelatine has dissolved, lightly stir to ensure it has completely melted. Pour the mixture through a strainer (I use a tea strainer) into a small, clean bowl and allow to cool for at least 10 minutes.

Add the cream cheese, erythritol and liquid stevia (if using) to the bowl of lime zest. Mix vigorously to loosen the cream cheese. Set aside.

In a larger, separate bowl, use a hand mixer to whip the double cream to soft peaks. Add the cream cheese mixture and the cooled gelatine mixture and mix well to combine.

It will stiffen quickly, so pour the mixture immediately onto the cooled base and smooth the top. Place in the refrigerator to set for 5 hours.

To serve, carefully lift the cheesecake out of the tin and peel away the parchment paper. Use a fine zester to grate the zest of the remaining lime over the top to decorate. Slice into 8 pieces and enjoy!

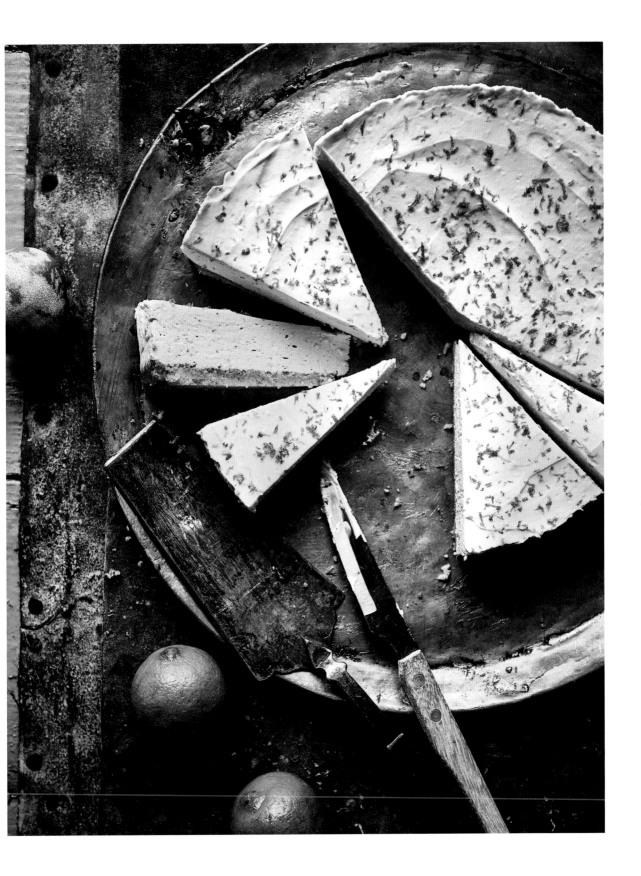

Coffee & Walnut Mug Cakes

I adore coffee-flavoured things, so this is great combo for a sweet treat to enjoy if the craving hits. You will love the texture the walnuts bring, and I like to go a step further by toasting them beforehand for maximum flavour. *Pictured on page 131.*

 2 MUG CAKES   **5m** PREP TIME   **5m** COOK TIME

CALORIES 587 | CARBOHYDRATES 5.7G | PROTEIN 15G | FAT 55G

25g (1oz) unsalted butter

2 teaspoons instant coffee granules

20ml (¾fl oz) double cream

1 large egg, whisked very well

30g (1oz) walnuts, chopped small, plus extra to serve (optional)

70g (2½oz) almond flour

40g (1½oz) powdered erythritol, sifted

1 teaspoon baking powder

2 tablespoons extra-thick double cream, to serve

Melt the butter in a small pan over a low heat. Set aside to cool (see Tip).

Use a very small bowl or ramekin to dissolve the instant coffee granules in one tablespoon of boiling hot water. Set aside to cool (see Tip). Place the melted butter, dissolved coffee, double cream and whisked egg in a bowl and whisk well to combine.

In the meantime, toast the chopped walnuts in a dry, non-stick pan over a medium heat until golden. Remove from the heat and set aside.

Place the almond flour, erythritol and baking powder in a bowl and use a clean, dry whisk to combine well. Tip in the egg-and-coffee mixture and mix well before folding in the toasted walnuts.

Divide this mixture between 2 greased ramekins or appropriately sized, microwave-friendly mugs and place one at a time in the microwave for 90 seconds. Remove carefully (they will be hot) and serve while still warm with a dollop of extra-thick double cream. If you feel fancy, you can decorate them with more chopped, toasted walnuts.

Cool the melted butter and the dissolved coffee slightly to avoid cooking parts of the egg when mixing.

Lemon & Poppy Seed Cupcakes

Lemon and poppy seeds are such a delightful combination! This recipe took a few trials to achieve optimum texture and flavour (leaving me with a ridiculous number of zested lemons in my refrigerator!), but I am pleased to say that the end result is lovely and, in fact, dead easy. *Pictured on page 130.*

 12 CUPCAKES   **15m** PREP TIME   **25m** COOK TIME

CALORIES 240 | CARBOHYDRATES 3.3G | PROTEIN 6.6G | FAT 22G

For the cupcakes

70g (2½oz) unflavoured coconut oil

4 large eggs

100g (3½oz) soured cream

130g (4¾oz) almond flour

25g (1oz) coconut flour

pinch of salt

1 teaspoon baking powder

1 teaspoon bicarbonate of soda

100g (3½oz) powdered erythritol

1 tablespoon poppy seeds

finely grated zest of 2 lemons

For the cream cheese frosting

270g (9½oz) full-fat cream cheese

2 tablespoons powdered erythritol, sifted

4–5 drops liquid stevia (optional)

finely grated zest of 1 lemon, to decorate

If you do not want the tops to darken too much, gently lay a sheet of kitchen foil over the baking tray after the first 10 minutes of baking.

Preheat the oven to 180°C/160°C fan/350°F/gas mark 4 and line a 12-cup baking tray with paper cupcake cases.

Melt the coconut oil in a small pan over a very low heat. Set aside and allow to cool slightly.

Crack the eggs into a large bowl. Add the soured cream and the cooled, melted coconut oil. Whisk well to a smooth, emulsified mixture.

In a second large bowl, combine the almond flour, coconut flour and salt. Sift in the baking powder, bicarbonate of soda and erythritol. Combine very well using a dry whisk to ensure everything is evenly distributed. Stir through the poppy seeds and lemon zest.

Pour the egg mixture into the dry flour mixture and mix thoroughly to combine. The batter is very wet, but don't worry; it will cook beautifully. Divide between the cupcake cases.

Place the tray on the lowest rack and bake for 10 minutes (see Tip). Then reduce the oven temperature to 160°C/140°C fan/325°F/gas mark 3 and bake for another 20 minutes (or until a cake tester comes out clean when inserted).

Remove the tray from the oven. Gently remove each cupcake case from the tray and set aside on a cooling rack.

While the cupcakes are cooling, make the frosting. Drain and discard any wateriness from the packaged cream cheese. Place into a bowl and whisk well, adding the erythritol and liquid stevia (if using) until you have a consistency that is easy to work with. Fill a piping bag fitted with a star nozzle and pipe the frosting on top of each cooled cupcake. Finish with finely grated lemon zest just before serving.

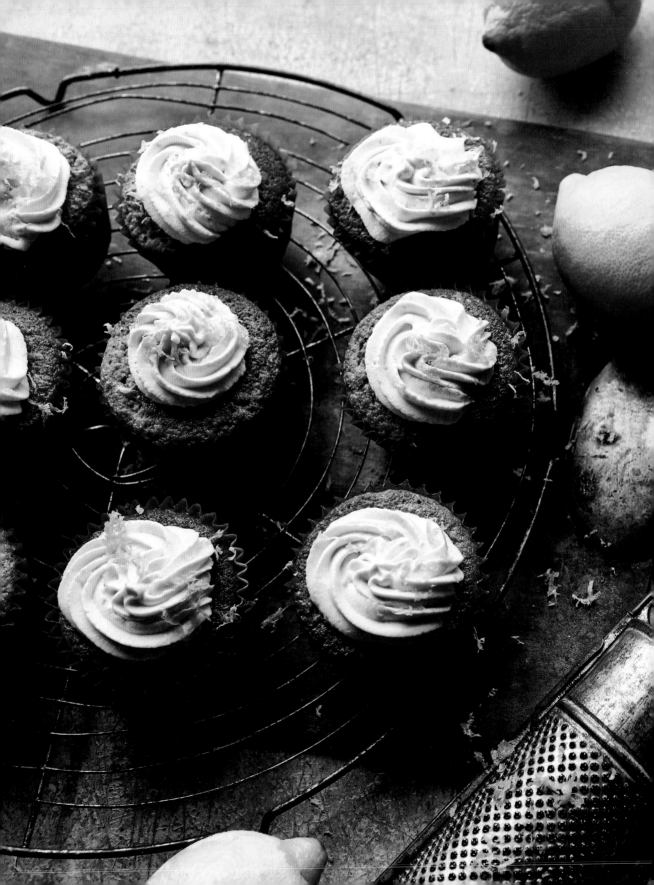

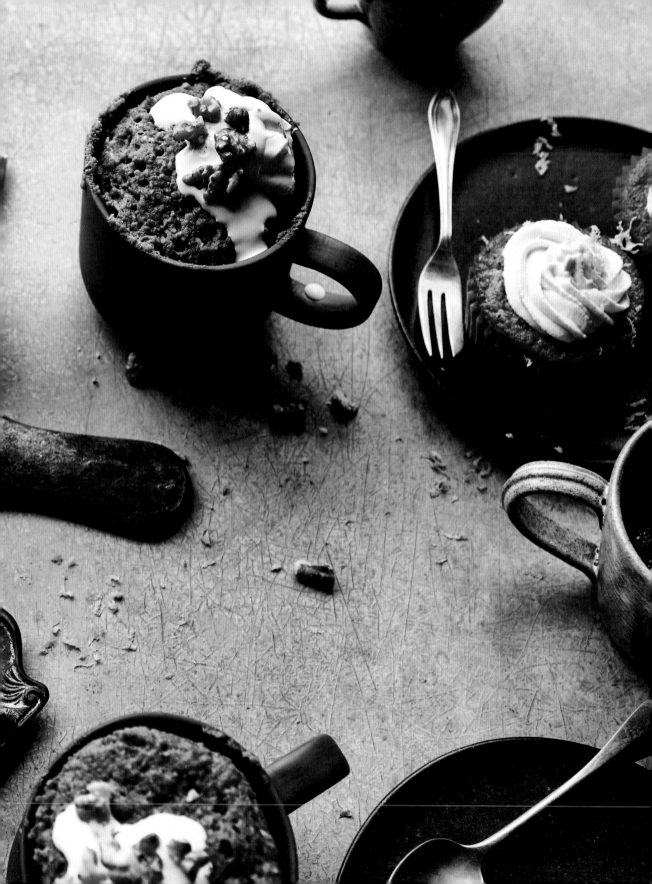

Chocolate & Raspberry Tart

I love the contrast of dark chocolate and sweet raspberries and thought this was a great way to pair them up. Not only is the pretty dessert decorated with fresh raspberries, but there are plenty hidden right there in the set ganache. Each slice of this dreamy treat comes in at only 5.4g carbs and your non-keto guests won't even know the difference! Use your favourite dark chocolate, but it should be 85 per cent cocoa for best results.

 8 SERVINGS **20m** PREP TIME **12m** COOK TIME **5hrs** SETTING TIME

CALORIES 390 | CARBOHYDRATES 5.4G | PROTEIN 5.8G | FAT 37G

For the base

120g (4¼oz) almond flour

30g (1oz) powdered erythritol, sifted, plus extra to decorate

1 tablespoon cocoa powder

50g (1¾oz) unsalted butter

For the tart

180g (6½oz) fresh raspberries

100g (3½oz) dark chocolate (85 per cent cocoa), broken into small pieces

200ml (7fl oz) double cream

50g (1¾oz) unsalted butter, diced small

I advise removing the tart from the refrigerator about 15–20 minutes before enjoying.

Preheat the oven to 200°C/180°C fan/400°F/gas mark 6.

For the base, mix the almond flour, erythritol and cocoa powder in a bowl. Gently melt the butter in a small pan over a low heat, then pour it into the almond flour mixture. Combine well and tip into a greased, loose-bottomed fluted tart tin (18cm/7in diameter). Press the mixture down to form an even, compact layer on the bottom and up the sides of the tart tin. Bake for 12 minutes, then remove and allow to cool completely on a cooling rack.

Once cooled, carefully remove the tart from the tin and place onto a serving plate or cake stand. Set a handful of the raspberries aside for decoration and slice the rest in half. Scatter the halved raspberries into the cooled tart case and set aside while you make the ganache.

Gently melt the chocolate in a non-stick pan over a very low heat. At the same time, gently heat the double cream in a separate pan over a low heat.

Pour the warmed cream into the melted chocolate and whisk well to combine. Immediately whisk in the small cubes of butter and watch the mixture become beautifully glossy. It if looks like your mixture has split or become grainy, add a tablespoon of boiling hot water straight from the kettle and continue to whisk. Pour the glossy, smooth mixture over the raspberries in the tart case and smooth it over.

Place in the refrigerator to set for at least 5 hours.

Just before serving (see Tip), decorate as you please with the reserved raspberries and dust over a little erythritol before slicing into 8 pieces.

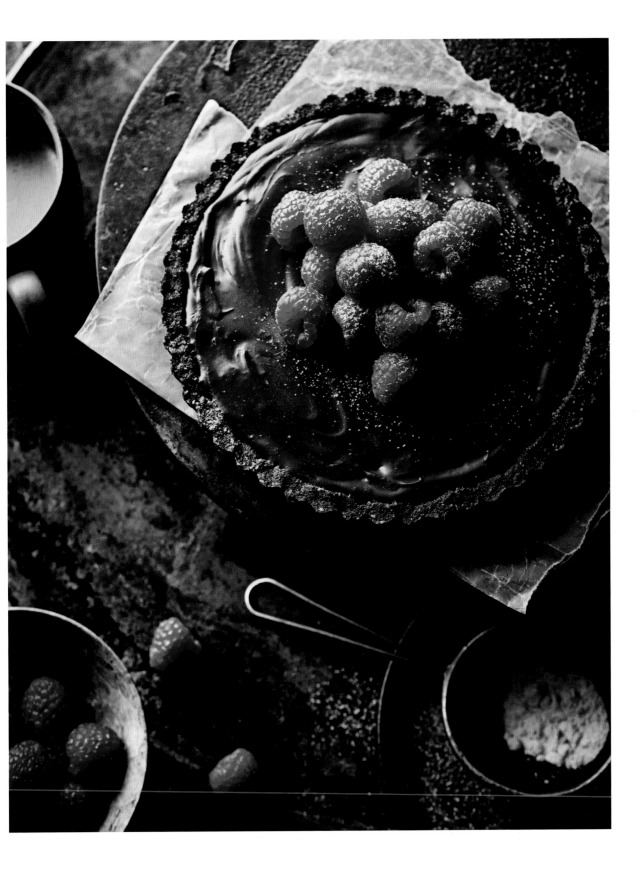

Double Chocolate Mousse

This is a decadent, sweet treat. With a little imaginative decorating using shaved or grated dark chocolate, it also makes a beautiful dinner party dessert to dazzle your guests. To ensure your mousse does not become gritty, allow the melted chocolate for the chocolate layer and the melted cocoa butter buttons for the white chocolate layer to cool before folding through the whipped cream. Remember that the mousse sets quickly so it needs to be spooned or piped into your chosen dessert bowls immediately after being made.

4 SERVINGS

30m PREP TIME

CALORIES 629 | CARBOHYDRATES 7.1G | PROTEIN 4.6G | FAT 65G

For the chocolate layer

100g (3½oz) dark chocolate (85 per cent cocoa), broken into pieces

220ml (7½fl oz) double cream

1½ tablespoons powdered erythritol, sifted

For the white chocolate layer

10g (¼oz) cocoa butter buttons

180ml (6¼fl oz) double cream

2 tablespoons powdered erythritol

3–4 drops liquid stevia (optional)

For the chocolate layer, start by melting 90g (3¼oz) of the dark chocolate in a pan over a very low heat. Set aside to cool.

Whip the double cream in a medium-sized bowl to soft peaks using a hand mixer. Add the erythritol and continue to whip to stiff peaks. Fold through the cooled, melted chocolate and immediately divide between 4 suitably sized dessert bowls or glasses.

For the white chocolate layer, melt the cocoa butter buttons in a small pan over a very low heat. Set aside and allow to cool.

Whip the double cream in a medium-sized bowl to soft peaks. Add the erythritol and liquid stevia (if using) as well as the cooled, melted cocoa butter and whip well. It will stiffen quickly, so spoon or pipe immediately over the chocolate layer.

Grate or shave the remaining dark chocolate over the desserts to decorate and store in the refrigerator until needed (see Tip).

If you decide to make these desserts ahead of time, remove them from the refrigerator at least 30 minutes before tucking in.

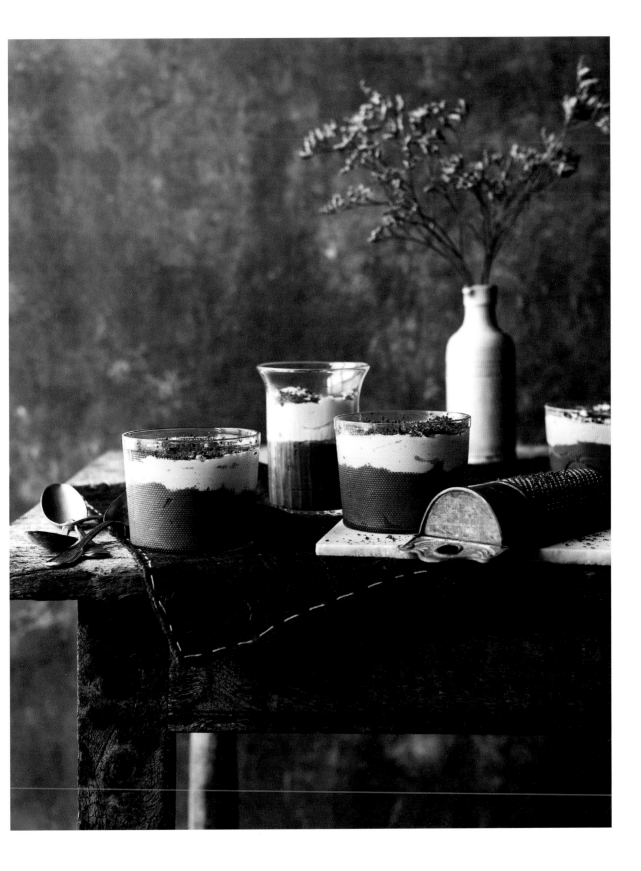

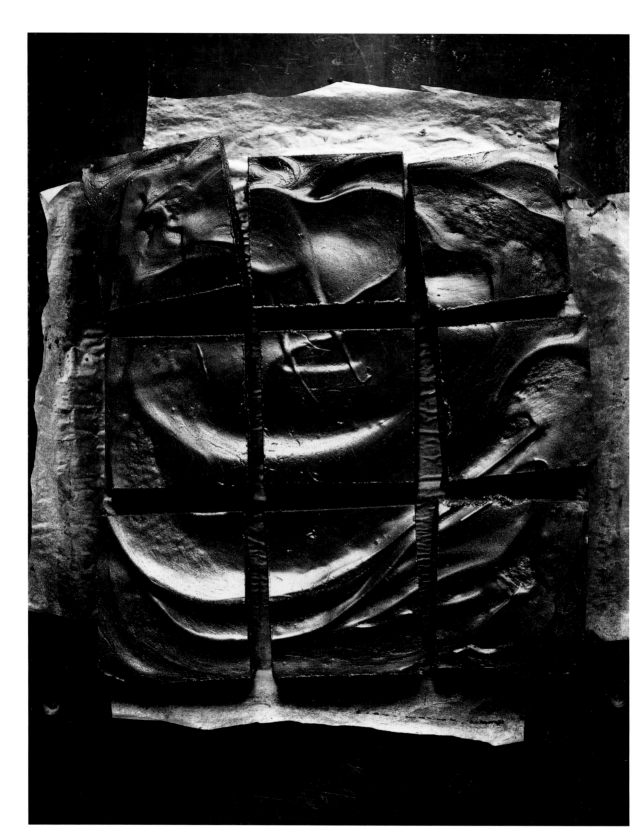

Decadent Chocolate Brownies

These brownies are my husband's favourite. He loves them as is, but sometimes heats them for a few seconds in the microwave and drizzles over a little double cream. They freeze really well, meaning it's easy to keep a treat on hand.

 9 BROWNIES   **10m** PREP TIME   **25m** COOK TIME   **3hrs** SETTING TIME

CALORIES 360 | CARBOHYDRATES 4.3G | PROTEIN 8.3G | FAT 34G

For the brownies

120g (4¼oz) unflavoured coconut oil

3 large eggs

4–5 drops liquid stevia (optional)

175g (6oz) almond flour

150g (5½oz) powdered erythritol, sifted

40g (1½oz) cocoa powder, sifted

For the ganache layer

50g (1¾oz) dark chocolate (85 per cent cocoa), broken into small pieces

50ml (1¾fl oz) double cream

2 teaspoons unsalted butter

Preheat the oven to 190°C/170°C fan/375°F/gas mark 5. Grease and line a square baking tin (approximately 15×15cm/6×6 in) with parchment paper.

Melt the coconut oil in a bowl in the microwave for approximately 45 seconds on medium heat and allow to cool before whisking in the eggs. Add the liquid stevia (if using) and whisk well to combine.

Combine the almond flour, erythritol and cocoa powder in a second bowl. Add the wet egg mixture to the bowl of dry almond flour mixture and mix well to combine. Tip the mixture into the prepared tin. Bake in the oven for 15–18 minutes or until a skewer inserted in the very centre comes out clean. (I always rotate the tin halfway through.)

Once done, place the tin on a cooling rack and allow to cool completely.

Meanwhile, make the ganache. Gently melt the chocolate in a non-stick pan over a very low heat. At the same time, gently heat the double cream in a separate pan over a low heat. Pour the warm cream into the melted chocolate and whisk well. Immediately whisk in the butter. The mixture should become beautifully glossy. If it splits or becomes grainy, add a tablespoon of boiling hot water and continue to whisk.

Remove from the heat and leave to cool for about 10 minutes, then pour the glossy chocolate over the cooled brownie cake and leave to set for at least 3 hours in the refrigerator. Once cooled completely, slice into 9 equal-sized squares. Store, covered, in the refrigerator (or wrap and freeze the individual squares). I advise removing the brownies from the refrigerator about 30 minutes before enjoying.

Almond & Cinnamon Ice Cream

If you love and long for ice cream, I think you should give homemade ice cream a try. With a little technical knowledge, it's actually very easy. Invest in an ice-cream maker, which will churn the mixture properly, and you are good to go! I strongly advise that you invest in a thermometer probe if you do not already have one. The egg in the ice cream base needs to be safely heated, but not overcooked, and there is little room for error here to avoid ruining the batch. Serve topped with roasted almonds if you want additional crunch.

10 SERVINGS | **20m** PREP TIME | **30m** COOK TIME | PLUS CHURNING AND COOLING TIME

PER 100G (3½OZ) – APPROX. 2 SCOOPS | CALORIES 382 | CARBOHYDRATES 3.5G | PROTEIN 7G | FAT 37G

For the roasted almond and cinnamon butter

300g (10½oz) raw, whole almonds

2 tablespoons powdered erythritol, sifted

2 teaspoons ground cinnamon

For the ice cream base

350ml (12fl oz) double cream

350ml (12fl oz) single cream

100ml (3½fl oz) unsweetened almond milk

1 vanilla pod, seeds scraped

3 large egg yolks

60g (2¼oz) powdered erythritol, sifted

4–5 drops liquid stevia (optional)

¼ teaspoon ground cinnamon

Ice-cream makers differ, but most household ones have a bowl that needs to be frozen solid before churning, so make sure you check the instructions and freeze the bowl first if needed.

For the roasted almond and cinnamon butter, preheat the oven to 180°C/160°C fan/350°F/gas mark 4. Spread the almonds out on a baking tray lined with parchment paper. Bake in the oven for 20 minutes, shaking and rotating the tray halfway through. Allow to cool slightly, then transfer to a mini food processor and blitz well to fine crumbs. Scrape down the sides of the bowl, add the cinnamon and erythritol and continue to blitz until the mixture starts to look very oily (or similar to fairly smooth peanut butter). Weigh out the 200g (7oz) you need for this ice cream recipe and keep the remainder in the refrigerator for another use (such as the Fat Bombs on page 123).

To make the ice cream, place the double cream, single cream and almond milk in a non-stick pan. Add the vanilla seeds and scraped pod to the pan. Add the egg yolks and whisk continuously over a gentle heat. Do not allow the mixture to rise above 70°C/158°F. This will ensure that the eggs cook through safely, but don't scramble –and this is why your thermometer probe is essential. Once this temperature is achieved, maintain it for at least 10 minutes.

Remove the pan from the heat and whisk in the erythritol, liquid stevia (if using) and ground cinnamon. Strain the mixture into a bowl using a fine mesh sieve, discarding the scraped vanilla pod. Whisk in the 200g (7oz) roasted almond and cinnamon butter and place the bowl in the refrigerator for at least 1 hour so the mixture can cool.

When you are ready to churn, set up the ice-cream maker (see Tip, left). Whisk your cooled ice cream mixture once more, then pour it into the ice-cream maker bowl. Churn according to the manufacturer's instructions (this takes approximately 30–35 minutes) and you will be left with a thick, creamy ice cream that is ready to scoop and eat or be placed in a suitable container and kept in the freezer.

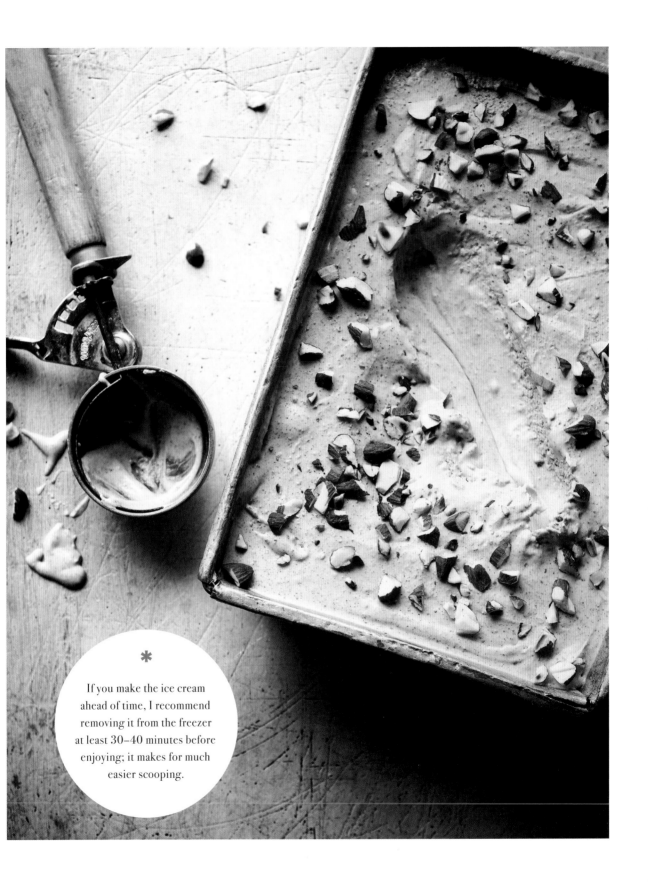

*

If you make the ice cream
ahead of time, I recommend
removing it from the freezer
at least 30–40 minutes before
enjoying; it makes for much
easier scooping.

Strawberries & Cream Lollies

These refreshing creamy lollies are so easy to make! I whip sweetened cream, incorporating plenty of air, then fold through partially mashed strawberries. I always have a batch of keto lollies in the freezer and the look on Mark's face when he sees them is simply unbeatable! Lolly moulds are readily available, and they are a great little investment. You can use your imagination to incorporate different fruits, like mashed blueberries or raspberries. I have at least 15 different combos in my arsenal, but I love this one the most!

6 LOLLIES | **20m** PREP TIME | **6 hrs** FREEZING

CALORIES 214 | CARBOHYDRATES 3.7G | PROTEIN 0.9G | FAT 21G

250g (9oz) trimmed strawberries, diced very small

250ml (9fl oz) double cream

3 tablespoons powdered erythritol, sifted

2–3 drops liquid stevia (optional)

Place the diced strawberries in a bowl and use the back of a fork to partially mash them.

Use a hand mixer to whip the cream and erythritol in a bowl to semi-stiff peaks. Fold through the mashed strawberries and liquid stevia (if using) and fill 6 lolly moulds (100ml/3½fl oz capacity) with the mixture. Since the mixture is firm, you will need to spoon it in a little a time and tap the lolly mould on the worktop to remove air pockets.

Place in the freezer overnight or for at least 6 hours. Remove from the freezer about 30 minutes before enjoying!

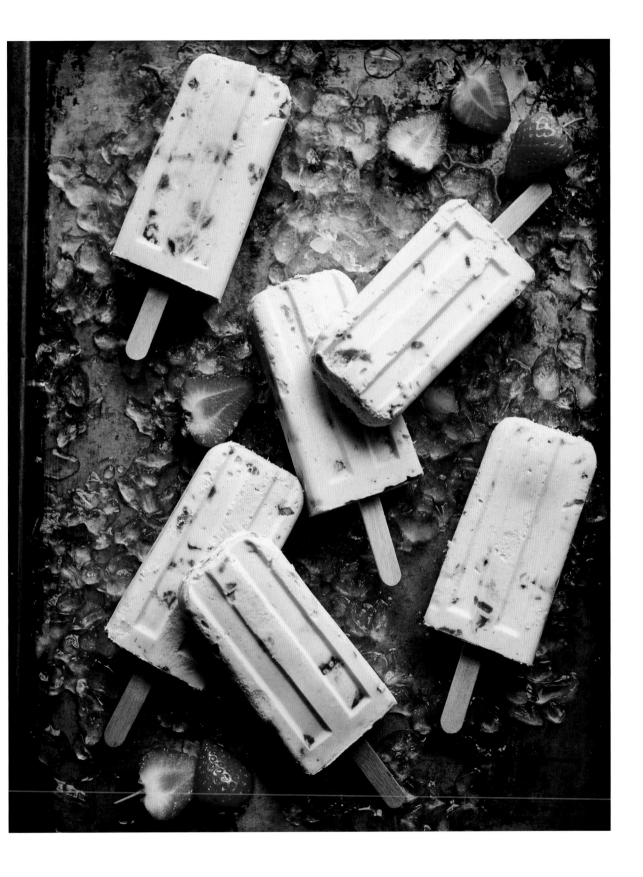

Index

UK/US Glossary

aubergine – eggplant
bicarbonate of soda – baking soda
baking tray – baking sheet
beansprouts – mung bean sprouts
clingfilm – plastic wrap
coriander – cilantro
courgette – zucchini
crisps – chips
double cream – heavy cream
frying pan – skillet
grill – broil/broiler
minced beef – ground beef
pak choi – bok choy
prawns – shrimp
rocket – arugula
single cream – light cream
soured cream – sour cream
spring onions – scallions

References

Abrams, Rami and Abrams, Vicky, *Keto Diet for Dummies* (Hoboken: John Wiley & Sons, Inc., 2019)

Atkins, Robert C, *New Diet Revolution* (London: Vermilion, 1999)

Noakes, Tim, Proudfoot, Jonno and Creed, Sally-Ann, *The Real Meal Revolution* (London: Robinson, 2015)

foodinsight.org/sugar-alcohols-fact-sheet/

foodstandards.gov.au/science/monitoringnutrients/afcd/Pages/foodsearch.aspx

greekgoesketo.com/ketosis-babies-untold-truth/

healthline.com/nutrition/are-vegetable-and-seed-oils-bad#section5

healthline.com/nutrition/modern-nutrition-policy-lies-bad-science#section1

healthline.com/health/oxidative-stress

medicalnewstoday.com/articles/262881.php

medicalnewstoday.com/articles/318652.php

paleoflourish.com/is-sesame-oil-paleo

psychologytoday.com/gb/blog/the-mindful-self-express/201302/why-our-brains-love-sugar-and-why-our-bodies-dont

thedaisygarland.org.uk/epilepsy-and-the-ketogenic-diet

nutritics.com

Recommended Reading

Abrams, Rami and Abrams, Vicky, *Keto Diet for Dummies*

Axe, Josh, *Keto Diet: Your 30-Day Plan to Lose Weight, Balance Hormones, Boost Brain Health, and Reverse Disease*

Fung, Jason, *The Obesity Code: Unlocking the Secrets of Weight Loss*

Nora Gedgaudas, *Primal Fat Burner: Going Beyond the Ketogenic Diet to Live Longer, Smarter and Healthier*

Noakes, Tim, Proudfoot, Jonno and Creed, Sally-Ann, *The Real Meal Revolution*

www.dietdoctor.com

www.zoeharcombe.com

www.thenoakesfoundation.org

Acknowledgements

Firstly, I want to thank my lovely agent Clare. I knew I was in good hands that first morning we met. To the team at Kyle: Judith, Jo, Florence, Gemma, Nic and especially my kind and patient editor Tara – thank you for turning my dream into reality. To Nicky, our designer – thank you for creating a beautiful book.

Maja and Olivia ... I am at a loss for words here. I had to pinch myself at every shoot to believe that what was happening was real. You both show sublime talent and integrity with your craft. Thanks also to Lisa and my assistant Lola; I simply could not have asked for a better team.

To the nutritionists, health coaches and doctors around the world who proofread and contributed to my manuscript: Gillian Harvey, Karine Ricard, Christina Oman, Dr Andrew Oswari (MD) and Dr Casey Cordial (DC, MS, DACBSP) – I am eternally grateful and deeply humbled that you volunteered your time to ensure I got the medical bits spot on. (I am better in the kitchen than I am at the science!)

Thank you to Lindy, Ollie, Emma and Annelise for ensuring there were no malapropisms (or 'Monniesms', as my loved ones call them) landing on my editor's desk; I am famous for using them! To all the recipe testers: Amanda, Angie, Cindy, Ellie, Janene, Joanita, Jules and Jason, Julie, Kim and Jay, Malcolm, Nicola, Pippa, Olivia and JJ, Stella, Sue and Brian – you helped me shape each dish to perfection. Your generosity of time and feedback was extremely valuable, thank you.

To Heston, Ash P-W, Papi, Big D, Shatton and Disco ... how fortunate I am to work with the best in the business! Thank you all for teaching me to push boundaries and be a better cook.

Saving the best for last, my darling Mark. You are the funniest man I know, a rock star at the *braai* and the best thing that ever happened to me. This is for you ...

Monya